T3-BQR-679

A PSYCHIATRIST'S VIEWS

ON SOCIAL ISSUES

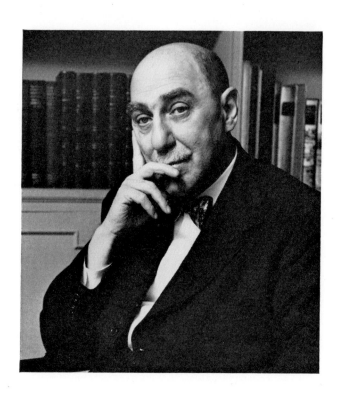

SOL W. GINSBURG, MD

A Psychiatrist's Views
on Social Issues

FOREWORD BY KARL A. MENNINGER, MD

INTRODUCTION BY WILLIAM C. MENNINGER, MD

COLUMBIA UNIVERSITY PRESS

NEW YORK AND LONDON 1963

Copyright © 1963 Columbia University Press

Library of Congress Catalog Card Number: 63-10913

Manufactured in the United States of America

CONTENTS

III.   The Practice of Psychiatry

PREFACE

THIS COLLECTION of the major scientific papers of the late Sol W. Ginsburg has been assembled for the benefit of social scientists, psychologists, social workers, educators, and theologians who are interested in the potential contributions of psychiatry to their several disciplines and professions. It should also help the growing number of psychiatrists who are becoming aware of the relevance of the social environment for the prevention and treatment of emotional disorders.

Although first and foremost a clinician, Dr. Ginsburg devoted a large part of his professional life to fundamental research on unemployment, occupational choice, and work, primarily as a member of the interdisciplinary team of the Conservation of Human Resources Project of Columbia University. He co-authored: *The Unemployed* (1943); *Occupational Choice: An Approach to a General Theory* (1951); and *The Ineffective Soldier: Lessons for Management and the Nation*, 3 volumes (1959).

The essays collected in this volume enable the reader to learn directly about Dr. Ginsburg's approach to major problem areas in the field of social psychiatry. They illustrate what he found useful in the armamentarium of psychiatry for probing more deeply into social conflict. They reveal why he found it necessary to reevaluate the basic assumptions of the mental health movement. And they demonstrate the fruitful interchange that can exist between clinical work in psychiatry and social research.

In the selection and arrangement of these essays, I have had the advice and counsel of Dr. John L. Herma, who was closely associated with Dr. Ginsburg throughout the later years of his life.

Except for "The American Family," these essays have been previously published. They are reprinted here with only minor editorial changes. A few deletions have been made and a few connective paragraphs added so that references in the original articles which have become out of date in the course of time will not interfere with the author's effective communication of his subject matter.

As Director of the Conservation of Human Resources Project of Columbia University, to which Dr. Ginsburg contributed so much, I am happy that I had the opportunity to collect these essays and arrange for their publication. Our association was much more than professional. We were cousins, but he was dearer to me than a brother.

ELI GINZBERG

January, 1963

FOREWORD

A WARM HEART and lively mind characterized Sol Ginsburg. His kind face, his radiant smile, his warm handshake, and his deep, reassuring voice marked him immediately as a friend, and a friend worth having. He had interest and concern in many fields of human life. For him psychiatry was more than a scientific discipline and a clinical activity; it was a way of understanding conditions of suffering and confusion and malfunctioning of many sorts including some not usually labeled disease. To some of his colleagues those social applications of psychiatric science seemed digressions and diversions; to Sol Ginsburg they were a glorious frontier of psychiatry.

Sol Ginsburg loved to teach. In 1948 and several times thereafter he came to the Menninger School of Psychiatry in Topeka as a visiting professor. Hour after hour during the day, and many times late into the night, he met with groups of resident physicians and faculty members. He listened, he counseled, he smiled, he corrected, he questioned, he declaimed. As is apt to be the case in such intimate and effective teaching, many areas and topics were touched upon besides the techniques of psychiatric diagnosis and treatment—philosophy, psychology, sociology, theology, literature, economics, and medical education.

Even more important than the new knowledge he imparted was the example he set. Before these young doctors stood a man, a man who was a teacher, a friend, *and* a psychiatrist. Here stood a psychiatrist of skill and experience who had joy in his work and a catholic interest in the whole human world. "This," they said to themselves, "is the kind of psychiatrist that I would like to become."

This collection of his written articles in the field of social psychiatry gives some hint as to the broad scope and kindly spirit of his thinking.

KARL A. MENNINGER, MD

INTRODUCTION

IT IS A DISTINCT honor and my pleasure to introduce to you, the reader, a collection of some of the more significant writings of the late Sol Wiener Ginsburg. In so many ways he was a remarkable person. He was a physician and a psychiatrist with a very unusual vision of the challenging problems in our social order. He had an amazingly broad scope of interest. He was a student all his life. Particularly was he sensitive to the values in life, his own and those of others. All of these qualities his close friends recognized. They will be obvious to those who read these essays.

Part of the satisfaction in writing these words is to recall with unusually pleasant memories my many and close contacts with Doctor Ginsburg between 1946 and his death in 1960. The first of these was a personal letter he addressed to me, without our ever having met, at the Office of the Surgeon General of the Army in Washington, D.C. It touched on a particularly sensitive spot in my military experiences. All of us in the Army and the Navy and the Air Force were so frustrated by our inability to accomplish what we thought we should. Perhaps we had been unfair in expecting much more help from our colleagues in civilian life. On the other hand, many of the psychiatrists in civilian life had also been aware of many deficiencies in our chosen field of endeavor. We were so short of manpower. There were a minimal number of opportunities for training the greatly needed professional personnel. The total amount of research was a fraction of what it should have been. This ferment of dissatisfaction was not unapparent in various ways. It was in the waning days of the war that Dr. Francis Braceland and Dr. Robert Felix and I appeared before the Council of the American Psychiatric Association to voice these frustrations and our needs for much greater help to meet the problems that confronted us in psychiatry.

Doctor Ginsburg's letter dealt with this sense of frustration of what we had been able to accomplish, or rather what we hadn't been able to accomplish. He challenged me to try to organize some of this dissatisfaction in a way that might bring some constructive results. I recall so distinctly my surprise in receiving this suggestion from Doctor Ginsburg. We did have many mutual friends but up to this point we had never met each other.

This noble discontent that stirred in the heart of Sol Ginsburg, and many other of our colleagues, resulted in the organization of the Group for the Advancement of Psychiatry in May, 1946. The structure of the organization was to be made up of committees of psychiatrists, each committee to be composed of men with a mutual interest in a particular area involving psychiatry—the psychiatric curriculum in the medical schools, the relations of psychiatrists and psychologists in their work, research in psychiatry, public education in psychiatry, and others. The committees were charged with the responsibility to seek information, collect data, consult experts in other fields that were related to their interest, and then to organize and present their findings in a form that could be helpful to others.

One of my own very special interests, perhaps prompted by the ineffective effort to prevent mental illness in the military service during the war, was how we could apply our clinical knowledge to social problems, including prevention. Sol Wiener Ginsburg was a natural person to head up this committee. For the first five or six years of its experience, Sol Ginsburg was chairman, and until he was made the president of the organization, continued as a member of that committee. Although I am not sure, I believe this was probably the first group of psychiatrists to consider systematically how those of us in clinical practice could contribute both towards the understanding and the solution of the social problems in our culture.

Doctor Ginsburg grew up in New York City, a metropolis with many kinds of social groups—racial, ethnic, religious, economic. Perhaps this, in part, provided the foundation for his later work and deep interest in social psychiatry. He knew from the immediacy of his own experience the extent to which cultural, social, religious, and economic factors affected the lives and behavior of people. His personal experience was fortified by the fact that he was a voracious reader all his life, and this brought him into intellectual and personal contact with the leaders of other disciplines, with many of whom he maintained an extensive correspondence.

There were other factors, though, that contributed to Sol's unusual perspective of life. He was brought up as a believing Jew and was very closely identified with his uncle, Louis Ginzberg, one of the greatest Jewish scholars of modern times. He held a deep conviction of the value of religion and ceremonial life in the building and maintenance of the mentally healthy personality. His security in his own religious belief and background helped many young psychiatrists of other faiths to reappraise their own reactions and feelings towards their religious upbringing and commitments.

Always Doctor Ginsburg was concerned with the recognition of the influence of the therapist's sense of value in the treatment of every patient. One of his most significant essays is "Values and the Psychiatrist." He constantly hammered on the theme that the psychiatrist who turned his back on the world outside could not really help his patients get well, for they, too, had to adjust to a real world in which the conflicts of values were constant and central.

Doctor Ginsburg was well grounded and trained as a neurologist—a field in which he made several important contributions. Early in life he acquired a fundamental respect for science as a method of inquiry. He went on into the private practice of psychiatry and found time not only to treat many people, but to carry on some important research, to do considerable teaching. Many of his essays deal with his pioneering efforts to apply his knowledge from clinical psychiatry to social problems. He regarded psychiatry as an exciting discipline but one that was hardly complete. Hence, his own conviction that the search for new knowledge and the improvement and correction of existing knowledge were essential. In the essay "Mental Health: Theoretical Assumptions," he did a bit of testing of the fundamentals in this field of psychiatry—and mental health. He spent his entire life helping people to attain better health, but he could not overlook the fact that the scientific underpinnings of the theory left much to be desired. Never did I know him to be defensive about this. Rather, he considered that criticism and inquiry would lead to the strengthening of this foundation.

With his cousin, Eli Ginzberg, a nationally recognized economist and social researcher, Sol became deeply interested in the study of the unemployed. He and Eli were responsible for starting one of the first truly interdisciplinary teams in the United States.

Although physical disability made it impossible for him to serve during World War II, his understanding and empathy for the impact of military life and stress on vulnerable personalities is reflected in his significant contribution to the three-volume study, *The Ineffective Soldier*. He and his colleagues also had broken completely new ground in their study *Occupational Choice: An Approach to a General Theory*. It is questionable whether any psychiatrist played a larger role in fundamental research in social psychology than did Sol Ginsburg during the decades of the 1940s and 1950s.

As the chairman of the Committee on Social Issues for the Group for the Advancement of Psychiatry, Doctor Ginsburg realized that great caution and circumspection had to be used in bringing what psychiatry had to offer to bear on the assessment and possible solution of important social issues. As the result, he sought aid from leaders in many other fields and they responded. In this process the members of that committee in GAP were able to get a clearer picture of their own strength and limitations in the broad field of social change. These were in turn passed on to the other members of GAP and to our psychiatric colleagues through the very excellent reports issued by that committee.

The fact that he could lead this team so well reflected his own basic approach and values—a conviction of what dynamic psychology had to offer, a belief that it also had much to learn, and basic honesty and humility. With it all, he was a superior psychiatrist in his clinical practice. His essay "Psychiatric Consultation in a General Hospital" suggests the contribution that psychiatry—as practiced by an individual like Sol Ginsburg—has made and continues to make in humanizing the diagnosis and treatment of patients.

This collection of essays demonstrates the important con-

tributions this man made by showing the interdependence
of social and psychological factors in mental health, in the
role of the psychiatrist in therapy, in the theory and practice of social work, in the illumination of key problems in
the social sciences and social policy.

It is my judgment that this book of essays should be of
enormous interest and concern to psychiatrists. In addition,
however, it has equal application to social workers, psychologists, social scientists—in fact, to all who are interested
in or committed to increasing knowledge and the applications of knowledge about man and his relationships. As one
reads them, one can feel the depth of Sol Ginsburg's personality—an affectionate, thoughtful person, and, at the
same time, a forceful leader, giving of himself without stint
that the world might be better—this was Sol's purpose in
life.

WILLIAM C. MENNINGER, MD

SOURCES AND ACKNOWLEDGMENTS

1. "Mental Health: Theoretical Assumptions." Ruth Kotinsky and H. L. Witmer, eds., *Community Programs for Mental Health.* Cambridge, Harvard University Press, 1955.
2. "The Neuroses." *The Annals of the American Academy of Political and Social Science,* March, 1953.
3. "Adjustment: Its Uses and Dangers." *Child Study,* 1955.
4. "Adolescence." *Child Study,* Winter, 1950–51.
5. "Values and the Psychiatrist." *American Journal of Orthopsychiatry,* XX, No. 3 (July, 1950).
6. "Religion and Psychiatry." *Child Study,* Fall, 1953.
7. "Cultural Factors in Social Work." National Travelers Aid Association, 1954.
8. "What Unemployment Does to People." *American Journal of Psychiatry,* XCIX, No. 3 (Nov., 1942).
9. "The Role of Work." *Samiksa,* VIII, No. 1 (1954).
10. "Work and Its Satisfactions." *Journal of the Hillside Hospital,* V, Nos. 3–4 (Oct., 1956): Israel Strauss Commemorative Volume.
11. "The American Family." Not previously published. Read at the Annual Meeting, Family Service of Westchester, Inc., Rye, N. Y., May 12, 1959.

12. "Troubled People." *Mental Hygiene*, XXXII, No. 1 (Jan., 1948).
13. "The Private Practice of Psychiatry." *Bulletin of the Menninger Clinic*, XIX, No. 2 (March, 1955).
14. "Psychiatric Clinic Practice." *American Journal of Orthopsychiatry*, XVIII, No. 2 (April, 1948).
15. "Psychiatric Consultation in a General Hospital." *Journal of the Mount Sinai Hospital*, XXVII, No. 4 (July–Aug., 1960).

I. Psychiatric Concepts

I. MENTAL HEALTH:

THEORETICAL ASSUMPTIONS

IT IS OVER half a century since the "mental hygiene" movement was initiated. Clifford Beers' courageous autobiography [1] was published in 1908; the National Committee for Mental Hygiene [2] was launched in 1909. The intervening years have seen an immense expansion in the number and variety of activities loosely subsumed under the term mental hygiene, and this essay will examine the goals toward which all this endeavor is directed and the theoretical assumptions on which it is based.

Beers' concern with mental hygiene (the actual phrase is Adolf Meyer's [3]) grew out of his own destructive experience as a patient in a mental hospital. Reflecting this point of departure, mental hygiene in the beginning was primarily concerned with valiant and essential efforts to improve the hospital care of the mentally ill. To do this it was necessary to uncover and document the appalling conditions in psychiatric hospitals, to arouse the public to an awareness of these conditions, and to mobilize community pressure on legislative and administrative bodies to improve and expand facilities.

This was a proper first task for the mental hygiene movement, and has been conspicuously successful. Whatever the defects in contemporary mental hospital care, and they are many and major, no one would deny that there has been tremendous over-all improvement in the past forty years. A great part of the credit for this improvement goes to the devoted members, both lay and professional, of the National Committee for Mental Hygiene and of the various state mental hygiene societies, many of them affiliated with it.

Activities directed toward improving the care of the mentally ill do not, of themselves, require a theoretical basis, and there was no concern, in the early years, with theory. Once the community's attention had been directed to the shocking conditions prevalent in mental hospitals and citizens of humanitarian bent had been enlisted in the effort to better these conditions, a "program" was almost automatically at hand.

It was not very long, however, before the mental hygiene movement began to shift from its preoccupation with the care of the mentally ill and to invade areas which (it was thought or, perhaps better, hoped) promised the fulfillment of the preventive goals of the work, implied from the beginning in the term mental hygiene.[4] With the development of modern medicine and public health measures, other hygienists had achieved great success in the prevention of physical ills; it was inevitable that analogies should be drawn and efforts made to apply similar concepts and techniques to mental and emotional illness.

A real problem is the impossibility of finding a stated program which can reasonably be considered authentic and representative. One looks first to the National Association for Mental Health, the only national body devoted entirely to this work; then to the numerous state and local mental health organizations with their varying programs; and finally to a host of other organizations and individuals engaged in what they consider mental hygiene activities. Differences in goals, approaches, and methods are many and often wide. Hence, when I speak of "the" mental hygiene movement and accept the self-designation of certain individuals as mental hygienists, I never mean to include *all* groups or individuals, or to imply any significant degree of uniformity. As a matter of fact, it is a serious problem when practically any trained, partially trained, or even untrained person can represent mental hygiene, but this problem is hardly unique to this field of professional activity.

Despite this difficulty, it is necessary, if for no other than rhetorical reasons, to speak of the mental hygiene movement as though it were far more uniform than it actually is. The programs of organized mental hygiene groups are undoubtedly much more conservative in their goals and aspirations than some of those which I shall discuss and attribute in this general way to mental hygiene. Yet it remains a fact that these goals are put forward eloquently by people of authority, repute, and wide influence.

What makes it even more difficult to speak in any inclusive sense of mental hygiene is the fact that it has become so much more than a group of organizational activities. By now, mental health has become a social goal and a cultural value.

The mental hygiene movement has invaded a field which is indeed far flung, at what may prove to have been too rapid a pace. As early as 1930 Wechsler [5] found it necessary to issue a warning: "Enthusiastic mental hygiene tells us that it is concerned with the prevention of mental deficiency, criminality, the psychoneuroses, the psychoses, anti-social traits, family unhappiness, divorce, prostitution, alcoholism, sexual perversion, epilepsy and other such simple matters." Almost from its beginning, the mental hygiene movement made bold and brave steps into unexplored areas, armed with few and often still faulty instruments.

The stimuli to such rapid growth were abundant. In the first place there was the great and challenging increase in awareness of the proportions of the problem—a rudimentary recognition of the huge cost in personal and economic terms of what has come to be looked upon as a modern plague. Soon we were to be repeatedly reminded that "one person in ten would spend some time in a mental hospital." What that experience would probably be like was burned into the mind by graphic accounts and photographs of neglect, mistreatment, and cruelty. Thus, the first move was to stimulate pity and to appeal to moral values.

In fact, the whole concept of mental health may rightly be said to have become a new and compelling value in our society. As early as 1925 Adolf Meyer [6] was led to this stricture:

There are two ways of being interested in health; the common one is that of making a list and plan of all things that are good and desirable in life and giving the best possible description of Utopia and of perfection with recommendations as to how to get there. The way of the worker in modern hygiene is that of making a survey of the actual activities and conditions, and then of taking up definite points of difficulty, tracing them to an understanding in terms of causes and effects and to factors on which fruitful experimental analytical and constructive work can be done. The first type leads mainly to moralizing; the second type leads to conscientious and impartial study and to constructive experimentation. It is one thing to study the problem of mental and moral health in the abstract and another to take up the definite points at which the human being is apt to fail and to trace them specifically to factors which can receive consideration in experimental creative work and in a constructive school program.

The tendency to utilize value judgments as a basis for mental hygiene activities [7] has increased over the years. Not only does it supply much of the impetus to work of this kind; what is probably more serious, it is rarely explicitly acknowledged and probably remains relatively unrecognized. Mental hygiene has become increasingly a social movement and, as Davis [8] has commented, "It possesses a characteristic that is essential to any social movement: namely, that its proponents regard it as a panacea." He continues, "Since mental health is obviously connected with the social environment, to promote such health is to treat not only particular minds but also the customs and institutions in which the minds function."

To document his contention, Davis quotes some embarrassingly sweeping statements on the goals of mental hygiene, and says, "So many similar statements can be found in mental hygiene texts, articles, and credos that these quotations are typical." [9] One of them is from Rosenau: [10] "The ultimate in mental hygiene means mental poise, calm judgment, and an understanding of leadership and fellowship— in other words, cooperation with an attitude that tempers justice with mercy and humility." Another quotation Davis takes over from Bromberg,[11] who attributes it to a prominent spokesman of the movement:

Mental hygiene . . . presents many wider aspects. Industrial unrest to a large degree means bad mental hygiene, and is to be corrected by good mental hygiene. The various anti-social attitudes that lead to crime are problems for the mental hygienist. Dependency, in so far as it is social parasitism not due to mental or physical defect, belongs to mental hygiene. But mental hygiene has a message also for those who consider themselves quite normal, for by its aims, the man who is fifty per cent efficient can make himself seventy per cent efficient. . . .

Thus, two pressing forces, both entirely understandable,

lead to intensification of mental hygiene efforts and magnification of mental hygiene goals: a sense of compelling need and an increasing group of devoted and socially motivated workers. In these circumstances, it is not surprising that effort has outstripped firm knowledge and that theory has been left far in the rear, regarded pretty much as an impediment to "progress."

Such values as democracy, cooperation, ambition, freedom, success, and happiness are to be found everywhere in mental hygiene writings;[12] as Davis[13] comments, "Mental hygiene, being a social movement and a source of advice about personal conduct, has inevitably taken over the Protestant ethic inherent in our society not simply as a basis of conscious preachment, but also as the unconscious system of premises upon which its 'scientific' analysis and its conception of mental health itself are based."

To be sure, conviction and devotion to a system of values is essential in any activity, scientific or otherwise, if it is to prove productive. But the mental hygiene movement has not been so much rooted in these values as it has flowered in them, without benefit of a sound body of scrutinized and validated facts.

One of the great theoretical lacks in mental hygiene activity seems to me to be that we do not have an adequate definition of mental health. This inevitably results in a confusion of goals and an uncertainty of means; it creates a situation like that of a hunter stalking an unknown prey with weapons which may turn out to be quite unsuitable. The notion of normality (the "normal mind," the "healthy personality," etc.) is based to a large degree and often solely on the value system of the author using the term; probably, much of the difficulty that has arisen in our efforts to agree on at least a working definition of mental health stems from this fact. It stems also from a lack of exact and scientifically determined criteria for mental health, which is even more serious.

Early attempts to define mental health simply equated it with an absence of mental illness. This largely begged the question, since, except for evidences of the most serious disease, there is no satisfactory definition of mental illness. The borderline between mental health and illness is vague. It even fluctuates from one cultural, socio-economic setting to the next.

As time went on, people concerned with mental hygiene activities no longer spoke of mental health solely in contradistinction to mental illness, but now vaguely equated mental health with "happiness," "success," "maturity," etc., etc. Inevitably such broadening of the definition has made understanding more difficult, expectations more unreal, and frustration and disappointment more likely.

A relatively simple, working definition of mental health would be most useful, even if it were not entirely "scientific." In my work in other fields, my co-workers and I have settled for some such simple criteria as these: the ability to hold a job, have a family, keep out of trouble with the law, and enjoy the usual opportunities for pleasure.[14] Although this statement is crude, admittedly incomplete, and perhaps even naïve, it does set forth the crucial characteristics of mental health in lay terms—without becoming involved in "scientific" complexities that are still not justified by the state of our knowledge.

The notion of applying public health concepts to the prevention of mental and emotional illness is admittedly attractive, and many have been beguiled by it. But a program for the scientific prevention of disease must depend in the first place on more or less exact knowledge of the cause of the disease and of the modes of its transmission, and on possession of means for eradicating the etiological agents. Unfortunately, few of these prerequisites are available to workers in mental hygiene.

It is true that we now have an immense body of knowledge about the development of some kinds of emotional illness, especially the neuroses and certain disturbances of behavior (psychopathies). This knowledge is widely used (though not always by any means exactly or appropriately) in mental hygiene activities; yet it still lacks the preciseness which would make it in any way comparable with our knowledge of the definite etiological agents that have been determined in those aspects of medicine which deal with physical illness. It is still largely so tentative and incomplete that the conclusions to be drawn from it are often disputed even by specialists in the field.

In other areas of mental illness lacks in our knowledge of causation are even more glaring. Thus, relatively little is known about the cause of psychoses except in the field of the so-called organic diseases (syphilis, alcoholism, psychoses incident to cerebral arteriosclerosis, etc.), and even in these diseases, the role of the less exactly defined and less well understood "personality" elements is increasingly emphasized.

As Wechsler [15] said in 1930 (and it is still true): "Sad as it is to make the confession, the fact remains that, despite accumulation of knowledge, the ultimate cause or causes of nervous and mental disease is unknown." Much more recently, in a symposium on the epidemiology of mental disorders, Knight [16] said: "[In the sense of tracking down a causal agent] I don't believe that there is an epidemiology of the functional mental disorder, because there is not now known any single causal agent of mental illness, and I would feel fairly safe in predicting that no single causal agent ever will be found."

The illuminating report of the conference at which Knight spoke makes abundantly clear that anything near an "epidemiology" of mental and emotional illness is as yet almost entirely lacking. The scope of the problem is implied by the fact that even this single conference touched on matters as diverse and complicated as delinquency, suicide, mental deficiency, neuroses, psychoses, alcoholism, and psychosomatic illness. I can heartily agree with Lindemann's reaction: [17] "We haven't quite mastered the epidemiological approach."

I do not think this failure represents only a lack of exact knowledge of causation. Perhaps, more basically, the nature of mental and emotional illness precludes an epidemiological approach. With few exceptions mental and emotional illnesses are not "due" to any one thing or even to a number of things in a strict etiological sense, but represent patterns of reactions to the myriad factors that influence an individual in a given social, economic, cultural environment. It is true that, in his earlier writing, Freud postulated that the neuroses were due to specific sexual seductions in childhood, but this notion of specific cause has yielded to the accumulation of experience and knowledge and is no longer tenable.

Current mental hygiene activities fall into four major groups: (1) efforts to increase and improve facilities for the care of the emotionally and mentally ill: (2) attempts to increase people's knowledge about emotional development and to implant in them "healthy" attitudes toward themselves, their children, their jobs, their associates, etc.; (3) attempts to make the mental hygiene point of view pervasive throughout an entire field (such as education or nursing); and (4) attempts to change or help change social conditions (as, for instance, bad housing)—in other words, attempts to manipulate the environment in ways to make it "healthier."

The results of efforts to improve services for the mentally and emotionally ill—through surveillance, criticism, and constructive citizen action—constitute one of the brightest pages in the history of the mental hygiene movement.[18] This is attested by, among other things, better medical, nursing, and attendant services in hospitals for mental disease; more effective commitment laws; improved hospital procedures and statistics; and the whole and important development of child guidance clinics.

Some time ago, Dr. George S. Stevenson,[19] Medical Director of the National Association for Mental Health, equated "the mental health program" with the care of the mentally ill unequivocally, and listed ten evils "that should not [befall people] in a civilized society"—all ten of them instances of inadequate or distorted handling of the mentally ill.

But as early as 1933 Dr. Frankwood E. Williams, a previous Director of the then National Committee for Mental Hygiene, voiced concern about confusion between treatment and other activities which might more reasonably be considered "preventive." According to Williams,[20] "except by arbitrary definition, none of these [therapeutic] activities, by the widest stretch of the imagination, can be called mental hygiene activities." I, too, strongly believe that it is necessary to attempt a sharp distinction between therapy and "mental hygiene." In my judgment, the perpetuation of a confusion between the two vitiates much of the strength of mental hygiene programs.

It occurs to me, in this connection, that the very terms mental hygiene clinic and mental health clinic perpetuate an anomalous concept and should be abandoned; clinical—that is, treatment—centers should be called what they are, namely, psychiatric. I realize that "public relations" reasons to the contrary may be put forward, on the ground that people would be frightened off from going for treatment if facilities were bluntly labeled psychiatric. To me, this contention seems fairly tenuous; should it prove to any degree true, the situation would at worst present an area for further educational efforts.

A second important group of mental hygiene activities is composed of efforts to change people's attitudes through various educational devices—providing people with new and accurate information about a whole variety of matters directly and indirectly concerned with mental and emotional health: information about growth and development, child-rearing, sexual relations, work and recreation, religion, panic reactions in civil defense, etc., etc. It is obviously of the greatest importance to have as clear an understanding as possible of the educational processes involved and of the efficacy of these efforts.

Dr. Nina Ridenour,[21] a distinguished and enthusiastic practitioner in the field of mental hygiene and the author of many highly regarded pamphlets widely used in its educational activities, asks,

What criteria do we have as to the effectiveness of our educational techniques? The sad answer is: None to speak of. The amount of wishful thinking which goes on with respect to educational methods is appalling. . . . A desperate need in this field is for research in educational methods. Without it, we shall continue to waste much effort and make many mistakes of which we are not aware. . . . The only really valid criterion of the effectiveness of any technique is: *Does it change human behavior in the desired direction?* And the answer to this we rarely know. We must therefore await some basic research.

An awareness of the problems involved in attempting to change attitudes has led Ridenour and others to insist that the material for which they are responsible combine sound psychoanalytic theory, sound principles of communication based on learning theory, and a firm knowledge of the uses of mass media. They also constantly test their materials in practice, if on a rather empirical basis, without definitive research techniques.

Unquestionably, one of the reasons workers in the mental hygiene field have shied away from recognizing the necessity to study the effects of programs is the great and acknowledged difficulty in evaluation. Yet it is my conviction that with the help of people trained in research the necessary techniques can and must be devised and applied. Otherwise, there can be no real security in any method or approach.

Most of the theory on which current efforts to improve attitudes are based is derived from social psychology. Practically all the relevant studies have dealt with attitudes in what one might call "sociological" areas, such as religion, capital punishment, interracial relationships. Optimism about changing attitudes stems for the most part from success in influencing such superficial attitudes as a food or cigarette brand preference. Relatively little psychological study has been done on changing attitudes more deeply rooted in the personality,[22] such as attitudes toward parents, siblings, children, self, persons of differing culture or race.

In the entire psychiatric and mental hygiene literature, I could find no attempt to consider the basic problem of attitudes and how they may be changed, or to evaluate the techniques designed to change them. It is especially curious that a field like mental hygiene, in which psychiatric knowledge has been the keystone, should seemingly have been so uncritical. All psychotherapists know how long and valiant is the struggle to help people change their attitudes, and one would have expected them to be especially skeptical about the whole armamentarium of such mental hygiene activities—even when they earnestly agreed with the goals. Apparently, however, it has simply been assumed that the attitudes of adults can be changed; that such change can be effected by lectures, motion pictures, dramatic playlets, etc.; and that a shift in attitude will be followed by changes in behavior. This has been accepted on faith, as it were, as part of a credo.[23]

Experienced and highly competent authorities question the notion that "ideas as such may serve as promoters of mental health." Thus, Zilboorg [24] contends that:

Even ideas about mental health cannot do much because ideas . . . are not movers of instinctual forces but rather their representatives. . . . Man's over-estimation of his own intellect has become combined with our recent over-estimation of psychiatry and thus led us into a methodological path which is extremely popular and just as extremely devoid of scientific validity or practical potentialities.

Zilboorg, of course, does not stand alone in this belief, and I count myself among those who agree with him.

It is perhaps a truism that mere information and exhortation, despite the best intent and effort, are often futile and may even be destructive. People learn only when their emotions are involved. To me, certain analogies to therapy seem implicit and relevant. I hardly need emphasize that no strict parallel is intended between therapy and educational procedures as ordinarily conceived. On the other hand, if we take, for instance, work with mothers in a prenatal clinic designed to "educate" them in sound principles of child care and to inculcate healthy attitudes toward pregnancy, delivery, and their offspring, we see at once a number of striking similarities to the therapeutic situation.

First and perhaps most important is the presence of an impelling motive for seeking help. In therapy this grows from a personal conflict, usually reflected in a symptom; in a prenatal clinic it grows from a desire to be a good and successful mother. Hence, in both instances, the individual is *ready* to accept help. Second, an atmosphere relatively free of the punitive and judgmental encourages complete frankness. Third, the mother-educator relationship, like the patient-therapist relationship, is characterized by acceptance and confidence and by reliance upon a strong, healthy leader. There are manifest differences in these relationships, and the transference situation in therapy encompasses a great deal more and is much more complex, but certain basic similarities surely exist.[25]

I am not especially impressed by the argument that no similarity between therapy and educational mental hygiene programs can be valid because the former deal with "sick" people and the latter with "healthy," or "well," people. The borderline between the two is tenuous, and it seems to me safe to assume that the difference between the "sickness" of patients and the conflicts of participants in these educational programs is not so great as to invalidate comparisons between the processes designed to help them. Naturally, there are differences. A young mother attending a prenatal clinic differs from a patient or even from a person with "bad" attitudes which one is trying to change. However, to deny any similarity would be to conceive of the pregnant woman as entirely free of unconscious conflicts and to assume no motivation for learning other than the conscious desire to be a good mother. This might hold true of an occasional mother, but it would certainly not hold for all, or, I presume, for most of those who attend such clinics or participate in similar educational projects.

All this would emphasize the great advantage, if not in fact the necessity, of making the effort to change attitudes take place in a "natural" life situation and at a strategic period on the life history, as in the instance of the prenatal clinic. In studies of interracial housing it has been found that attitude change is maximally facilitated in the usual life situations of the tenants (the laundry, the bingo game, etc.). Kris[26] has emphasized that the problem of the methods of education has become more complex as a result of more recent psychoanalytic investigations and developments. He says: "Few if any clear-cut rules can be established: rather, every discussion of the handling of the means of education must take into account a multitude of developmental factors."

No extended mention has been made in this discussion of the content of the material used by mental hygienists in their effort to impart information and influence behavior. Obviously, this is of the greatest importance and represents an area in which there has been considerable discussion and thought. In general, materials borrow formulations, more or less as they stand, from psychoanalytic theory and practice.[27] This has been a not unmixed blessing.

At one time, education, especially at the nursery school and primary school levels, attempted to use a whole array of theoretical formulations taken over from psychoanalysis —only to discover that the application of such formulations was exceedingly complicated, and that even the soundest theory could not be taken over wholesale and applied uncritically, without adaptation.

To take a single example, teachers and parents were taught (persuaded) that permissiveness is, of itself, an ideal goal and one to be aimed for in all situations.[28] I need not remind you how futile, in fact destructive, much of such effort proved. On the theoretical side, the concept of permissiveness that was absorbed neglected the important ego-building functions of frustration and deprivation (discipline). On the practical side, it implied a way of dealing

with children that is well-nigh impossible, and so it frequently created conflict, doubt, self-recrimination, and
guilt on the part of parents, especially mothers.

Other examples come quickly to mind. The compelling
advantages of breast-feeding, for instance, were once widely
taught. That bottle-feeding could be occasioned by pressing reality needs, such as the necessity for the mother to go
to work, was for a while practically lost sight of in favor of
more beguiling theoretical considerations. We thus created
an immense burden of guilt in the mother who could not
nurse her baby. Only now are we busily tempering the
breast-feeding doctrine, admitting that modifications and
even failure to nurse need not necessarily result in any,
much less permanent, damage to the child.

Hoffer,[29] in an important and well-considered paper, emphasizes the immense complexity of attempting to apply
psychoanalytic insights directly to education, and the
hazards involved, even though the theory itself be sound
enough. For instance, he holds the drawbacks of psychoanalytic sex education to be caused not by an erroneous
application of analytic principles but by too rigid application of the results of adult analyses. And this stricture may
be extended to various other attempts to use psychoanalytic
insights directly in education. It is not for lack of sound
theory that education has encountered difficulties, but
rather because it has attempted, prematurely, to apply such
theory to too wide a range of problems, and to utilize it too
avidly and too uncritically. The theory was almost entirely
developed as a result of the observation, in therapy, of disturbed (sick) children and adults, and there are obvious
limitations in the application of knowledge gained from
study of failures in adaptation, the sick, in giving guidance
to the experience of the well.

Incidentally, we have only begun to acquire a usable

body of knowledge of the processes of development in the so-called normal child. Up to now, the direct observational study of children, either well or sick, has not proved so rewarding as was originally anticipated, but has rather served merely to confirm hypotheses established by reconstructing material gathered in the analyses of adults. However, we have good reason to hope that such study will in the future supply the data necessary to complete certain analytic principles and offer important contributory insights. Studies of familial settings, knowledge growing out of increased experience in residential treatment centers, and additional analytic study of normal children will add to a body of theory from which educational material may be more securely developed. But at present, the data we have are not sufficiently complete to enable us to be as confident as we would like about the advice we offer parents, teachers, and others.

What might be called the mental hygiene point of view sometimes pervades large portions of a field. This is most clearly illustrated in nursery school and primary education.[30] Vigorous and persistent efforts are being made to render this point of view similarly pervasive among professional people who play key roles at strategic times in the lives of individuals: teachers in general, the clergy, physicians (especially pediatricians and obstetricians), nurses, and, of course, social workers.[31] These efforts are marked by varying degrees of skill and thoroughness, and they rest on the same tenuous grounds as do efforts to change attitudes by educational measures, discussed above. But over-all they represent one of the most important and useful mental hygiene approaches. They are based on the entirely valid idea that members of these professions exercise great influence on others at certain crucial stages in their lives and in circumstances which are especially suitable for reconstructing and, if need be, redirecting entrenched feelings, orientations, and notions.

Still another group of mental hygiene activities are those in which broad social problems are discussed and social action to influence and change existing institutions (social reality) is recommended.

Lawrence K. Frank [32] has said:

It may be that many psychiatrists, because of the very nature of their clinical training and their preoccupation with concrete individuals, feel either indifferent to or baffled by any proposal [to translate knowledge of the innumerable ways in which human functioning can be disturbed or diseased over into a constructive program of redirecting the many aspects of human living, city planning, housing, nutrition, recreation, working conditions and the like, not only to prevent disease, important as that is, but to foster vitality and well-being throughout the population].

He adds that "such a proposal may appear so remote and perhaps so fantastic that many will believe it utterly Utopian and absurd," but expresses eloquently his own conviction:

If the new understanding of man's origin and development, of his immense capacities and, above all, of the amazing flexibility of human nature and its patterning by social life and culture, have any social significance they point to the realization that . . . he can, if he will, take charge of his destiny and begin to create the kind of culture and the kind of group life that is dedicated to human needs and values.

Although Frank is not speaking explicitly of mental hygiene, I have quoted him at length since his proposal is closely akin to, if indeed not identical with, much current thinking in this field. To say the least, such ambitious aims for mental hygiene stand in sharp contrast to the relatively modest goals and devices of therapy and education we have been discussing. I should hesitate to say they are beyond achievement, even allowing for the stark, bitter realities which confront our world. I should only say that we are still almost entirely without the theory and techniques which would make such aims translatable into a program for here and now. Moreover, incalculably great forces of greed, reaction, and ignorance stand opposed. I am inclined to agree with Whitman,[33] who says in relation to local community planning for mental health activities: "Horizons and vision may be limitless but tangible progress can be obtained only by breaking down the problem into discernible and well-defined areas of activity."

No one can deny that we desperately need a new concept of social living, and Frank's sense of urgency is understandable and appealing. Positive ideas of mental health, of family and group living, of freedom from prejudice and hatred are sorely needed. Moreover, it is perfectly true that the great reforms in the world did not wait on theory; there can be no criticism of those who, impatient with our plodding ways and lack of progress, envisage bold new steps.

However, in discussing the application of psychoanalytically rooted methods to everything from medicine, public welfare, education, management, and personnel practices to "unhappiness" and, "even, 'lack of luck,'" Kris[34] has recently warned that "at the threshold of this brave new world it seems appropriate to halt and raise the question: How well is science equipped to meet the tasks with which it is confronted, tasks set by society, in an age of rapid social change? Let me anticipate what I think is the answer—I believe there is some danger that the demand may outgrow our supply of firmly established knowledge, and that inferior products may temporarily 'swamp the market.'"

To be sure, psychological theory recognizes the baneful influence of such social phenomena as unemployment, bad housing, and discrimination against minority groups. It emphasizes (although it cannot quite document) the ways in which social reality patterns the conditions which lead to either satisfaction or frustration for the individual, and how it influences the kind and degree of self-expression and self-fulfillment he finds possible.

From such "facts" as these, the inference is drawn that anything which is part of destructive social reality makes for bad mental health and, further, that attempts to ameliorate such conditions fall rightly within the province of mental hygiene. Even if the "facts" were more firmly established, the inference would require the most careful scrutiny. I believe this whole area of mental hygiene activity represents another illustration of the way in which theory, often still tentative and incomplete, is used to implement perfectly good (meaning that I share them) value judgments.

It may be instructive at this juncture to examine "the principles of mental hygiene" as set forth by one school of thought. For this purpose I have chosen the contributions of the distinguished British psychiatrist H. V. Dicks, a devoted and experienced worker in this field.

Dicks [35] proposes that mental health be conceived as a new value in our world, "a new means of conquest of another dimension." He continues: "I believe that 'mental health' is an emerging goal and a value for humanity of a kind comparable to the notions of 'finding God,' 'salvation,' 'perfection,' or 'progress,' which have inspired various eras of our history, as master values which at the same time implied a way of life." He believes that "some of the attributes of a secular priesthood or therapeutae are attached to us," that "we have in our hands keys capable of unlocking human treasures perhaps greater than those which the atomic scientists have now, for good or ill, put at the disposal of ambivalent, anxious human beings."

His basic premises are these: [36] that the greatest single factor in the breakdown of an individual's mental health is "failure in human relationships"; that, aside from genetic factors, we find "etiology enough for the incidence of neurosis and allied disorders in the stresses and failures of human relationships"; and that "the task of thorough treatment of even the relatively benign psychoneuroses and milder character disorders is a time-consuming procedure beyond the powers of a much larger and better equipped cadre of specialists than is likely to come into being in a measurable time."

"For this reason alone," he says, "concentration of our man power on prophylaxis is essential," and by "prophylaxis" he means "not merely early treatment of established trouble," but *the creation of a social climate which favors good adjustment*" (italics mine.) [37] For him, the prescription for mental health is, in essence, "the simplest":

It consists in the protection and development at all levels of human society of secure, affectionate and satisfying human relationships, and in the reduction of hostile tensions in persons and groups. It is the championship of love and the elimination of hate in human affairs, with all the connotations and implications which these two concepts carry in the light of half a century of psychodynamic experience and research related to the fate and permutations of affect.

Dicks begins his consideration of what he calls "general mental hygiene" with the statement of a conviction which is implicit in much mental hygiene activity, but which is, unfortunately, seldom so frankly spelled out:

. . . much of the responsibility for promoting the health of a society lies not in the hands of its medical services but only within the scope of social practitioners: politicians, local and national, managers, teachers and other leaders and legislators of human groups.

Nevertheless, he holds that:

. . . it is mainly from informed medical and psychological opinion and advice that advances in the prophylaxis of mental disability and the promotion of good mental health are likely to flow into the counsels of social action.

He holds that psychoanalytic formulations must constantly be woven into an understanding of the social climate.

In this connection, Jahoda's [38] caution bears repeating:

The study of social issues should never be the exclusive concern of one branch of the social sciences. Such unilateral approaches lead to unconvincing theories about social issues. Wars cannot be explained by psychoanalytic theories of aggression alone; the behavior of one nation cannot be described satisfactorily by treating it as if that nation were a psychoanalytic patient on a couch.

For Dicks, as for others who share his perspective, it is plain that:

it would be rash to draw the line of prophylaxis of mental disorder at any given point and say: this is the legitimate boundary of medicine—beyond it lies politics. It is not the province of mental hygiene when a harassed young father in Kent has to leave his pregnant wife and two little children in "Bomb Alley" to join the Army, because a group of aggressive psychopaths in Berlin or Timbuctoo have seized power through exploiting the paranoid anxieties of their fellow-countrymen and are proceeding to translate those anxieties into invidious reality in war. Which is more ill: the young man who under such conditions develops an anxiety state or the political organization of the world which demands from him and extols as laudable such conflicts of motivation? And can we help his life if we cannot change society?

From such a statement we can discover the full scope of what Dicks envisions as the task of mental hygiene: "It is no less than the effort to change society."

The tools he proposes to use stand in bewildering contrast.[39] The measures he suggests turn out to parallel familiar mental hygiene programs, following the familiar application of psychoanalytic principles to child-rearing. (Here Dicks' own caution is worthy of note: "How can any rule of thumb guidance be given to millions of our parents, themselves members of our society which we have scarcely begun to study in psychodynamic and comparative terms?") Freudian principles are to be basic. First emphasis is to be on the family ("Pride of place in any mental hygiene programme must be assigned to the family") and the second on "education."

As "agencies of mental hygiene," Dicks relies on (1) teaching large numbers of young mothers and fathers "the delight, interest and techniques of fostering the natural development of their infants"; (2) enlisting the cooperation of teachers at every level, and furthering their (the teachers') education in sound principles of child growth and development ("the aim of the child guidance services of any given area should be to penetrate more and more into the community and there deal with incipient troubles while they are still problems, before they have become breakdowns"); (3) using the family doctor, the school medical officer, and the pediatrician "to accelerate the tempo of acceptance of psychological principles in home, school and community"; (4) establishing counseling centers for families, which would not only be the seat of the child guidance work but which would also offer skilled advice and social help to adults (on legal and vocational problems, housing, and so on.) At best, none of these should be identified with strictly medical services, "let alone have an overt psychiatric label." Special mental hygiene services are to be offered handicapped children, adolescents, ex-servicemen, bereaved persons, menopausal women, the aged, and industry.

If Dicks' extravagant expectations for changing the world and his vastly oversimplified ideas about world affairs, politics, social reform, etc., are left out of account, his actual program proves simple enough and remarkably similar to those of many state and local mental hygiene organizations, with their much more modest expectations.[40] To me, the supposition that Dicks' program, even if it were possible to carry it out to the fullest, could produce the new world he envisions, seems utterly naïve. Worse, such a concept would alienate many people from practical mental hygiene activities; disappointment and frustration would be bound to follow pursuit of such an impossible goal, and limited resources would be wasted in quest of the unobtainable.

Let me make myself entirely clear. I do not regard the complicated fields of political, social, and economic theory and practice as mere offshoots of psychiatric knowledge. Neither do I think that psychiatry is at present in any way equipped to make a frontal attack on adverse social realities. This does not mean that I think that those who are skilled in and knowledgeable about mental health activities have no role to play in efforts to ameliorate the conditions of life that are known to impinge deleteriously on the social and emotional functioning of large numbers of human beings.

I have noted above that psychological theory recognizes the baneful influence of such social phenomena as unemployment, bad housing, and discrimination against minority groups. In the light of the value system to which they adhere, responsibility rests upon all mental hygienists to speak out from the vantage point of their special competence whenever opportunity arises for constructive social action in regard to any such evils. The value of expert testimony to the ill effects of segregation on personality development and social functioning has already proved itself. For the field of mental health to attempt to teach the other disciplines that study social phenomena how to deal with them would be presumptuous; for it to fail to contribute what it can on the basis of its special knowledge would be irresponsible.

The mental health movement can point to the harmfulness of certain social conditions, but it is not expert in their amelioration. Its greatest helpfulness may lie through a program of research to discover more precisely than is now known the bearing of particular social conditions upon individual development and functioning.[41] For example, mental and emotional ill health will not be wiped out with the elimination of the slums, but the more precisely the harmful role of the slums is defined, the more realistic will be the methodologies for dealing both with the slums and their emotional consequences. This would clearly be the task of many disciplines, and not of those related to mental health alone.

In sum, I think it may be said in all fairness that the first need of the mental hygiene movement is to make a realistic appraisal of its assets, limitations, and goals. This would entail a critique of whatever theoretical knowledge is now available, an accounting of techniques solidly based on this knowledge, and an evaluation of these techniques as instruments for achieving goals tentatively accepted as valid. It is important always to recognize the dangers in outstripping available knowledge, and to study the wisdom and efficacy of activities under way.

A correlative need in the field is to clarify ideas about what training for this work should be. Obviously, no one discipline can ever hope to encompass all the needed knowl-

edges and skills. The weaknesses in the usual interdisciplinary approaches are well known; often they result in a
confusion of highly specialized language and conceptualization, with no real integration. Ideally, a mental hygienist
should be trained in psychology and psychoanalysis, sensitive to the problems of community relationships, and skilled
in group techniques and in the techniques of mass communication. Such training may well grow out of some modification of the education for psychiatric social work, which
at first glance, at least, seems the most suitable jumping-off
place.

This description of the mental hygienist of the future
serves to emphasize the fact that, generally speaking, mental
hygiene activity is now carried on either by people who
are not specifically trained at all or by those who are trained
in one area but who lack knowledge and skills in others
which are also highly essential. Well-trained psychiatrists
and psychoanalysts speak on mental hygiene without any
knowledge of education or the techniques of mass communication.[42] Any clinician writing on mental hygiene must
acknowledge the limitations which his training and daily
practice impose on him. The therapist's job is to help an
individual; such concepts as a "sick society," which seem
to have gained wide acceptance in the field, are relatively
new and remote to him.

On the other hand, educators who engage in mental hygiene activities often use psychiatric and psychoanalytic
theory and facts with no real awareness of their meaning
and implications. The corrective is a long way off. It will
ensue only when a satisfactory training scheme has been
devised and put into practice.

We need constantly to strengthen the hands of those who
are actively engaged in mental hygiene work. I believe this
can best be accomplished by study, research, self-criticism,

and surveillance of efforts, and by a frank facing of inadequacies and lacks. This is the hallmark of the scientist. The goal must be to transform this whole variegated body of activities and knowledge into a scientific discipline. To do this will not require any surrender of values, but only a reformulation of goals, expectations, and means.

2. THE NEUROSES

THE EMOTIONAL illnesses which are called the neuroses, or sometimes the psychoneuroses, form a highly variegated group of conditions, not easily defined or classified, and of a frequency at present quite beyond statistical reckoning. They are, as we shall see, illnesses of the gravest moment to the individual, the group, and the economy.

The first stumbling block in any attempt to determine the scope of the neuroses is the matter of definition. To define adequately a neurotic condition depends in its essence on a usable and acceptable definition of normalcy, a task of almost insurmountable complexity.

In the usual run of organic illness, the problem is, all things considered, relatively quite simple; for most of such disease processes there is a known, identifiable cause, a recognizable syndrome (a collection of symptoms and accompanying discernible evidences of malfunction), and a change in tissue structure or physiological functioning, demonstrable either by such devices as X-ray examination or studies of the chemistry of the blood and of the morphology of its cellular elements, or by actual microscopic examination of tissues.

In emotional and mental illnesses this is almost never the

case; even in the so-called major mental and emotional illnesses, such guides to detection and diagnosis are almost entirely lacking. Even statistical norms are lacking to help us in our search for a definition. A norm of sorts can be established for such things as height and weight, body temperature, the basal metabolic rate, and the chemistry of the blood. Such norms, however, are practically impossible to establish for character traits, modes of behavior, moods, patterns of thinking, and interpersonal relationships, which are all the very essence of a definition of normal for mental and emotional health.

Obviously, any estimate of normal must consider such variables as the culture or subculture in which the individual lives, the socioeconomic status, age and sex, and such even less tangible variables as the religion and the value system of the individual. Of equal importance is the perspective and value system of the person who is attempting to supply the definition of normal. "Normal" is a purely relative term, and short of the extreme deviations found only in conditions outside the scope of this discussion, the definition here used will reflect the beliefs and values of the observer as well as the observed.

Space limitations preclude a thorough exploration of this problem. I can only offer as background for a discussion of those deviations from normal with which I am to be concerned a rough working definition of normalcy, which has been used for years by the members of Columbia University's "Conservation of Human Resources" project: To be "normal" is to be able to hold a job; have a family; not get in trouble with the law; enjoy the usual opportunities for pleasure; and be free of anxiety or symptoms which would prevent one's usual round of duties and commitments.[1]

Such timeworn clichés as "Everybody is a little crazy" or "There are as many nuts outside as inside the asylums" suggest the common recognition of the fact that the borderline between normal and "sick" is indeed vague and ill defined. It is not accurate, of course, to say that everyone is "neurotic" if that term is to have any usefulness. But two things can probably be said with considerable validity.

First, all individuals possess what has been termed a "neurotic potential," which means that under certain circumstances everyone will experience feelings and display behavior which may be quite accurately termed neurotic (reflected in the Army's now familiar contention that "every man has his breaking point").

Second, everyone has some quirk of behavior, some habit of thought, some conflict in emotions, which *of itself* is of small consequence but which, theoretically at any rate, may be considered abnormal. An increase in the intensity of any such pattern of behavior or thought, or the combination of a number of such deviations, may lead to a clinically significant neurosis.[2] The executive who must have all his pencils neatly and freshly sharpened before he can begin work; the housewife made unnecessarily and often acutely uncomfortable by an unemptied ash tray or an unexpected guest; the compulsive smoker; the incessant doodler—these and many other such attitudes and patterns of behavior familiar to each of us in others and, on a moment's reflection, in ourselves, illustrate this point.

And it is not only the qualitative boundaries for neurosis that are difficult to establish; quantitative estimates are no more readily available or more exact. These days it is usual to quote as a ready and presumably reliable index of the extent of mental and emotional illness in the population the now familiar statement that about a million men were rejected for service in the armed forces because of such difficulties, and that for the same reasons about a million more men had to be prematurely separated from the services. Although these figures [3] are far too general and inclusive to have statistical validity, it can certainly be said that they indicate a wide distribution of such illness throughout the population.

In contrast to other illnesses, there are no available figures for the incidence of neurotic illness in the general population. Experienced practitioners of medicine will often say, "More than half the patients I see are neurotic"; but obviously such figures have merit only as impressions, and cannot command serious attention as statistics.

Strecker estimates that 75 per cent of all patients consulting the general practitioner have psychiatric disturbances, of which 5 per cent are psychotic, while the others have a whole array of mental and emotional problems, many of which are complicated by the presence of organic illness.[4] Similarly, McLean reports that 27 out of 100 consecutive patients admitted to the medical services of the University of Chicago outpatient clinic were found to be neurotics, 23 had questionable organic illness, and only 50 had clear-cut organic illness.[5]

It has been variously estimated that from 10 to 20 per cent of all patients admitted to general hospitals in this country have a neurotic illness and that about an equal number present some complicating emotional element in an organic illness.[6] In an important study of 450 admissions to the medical and surgical wards of The New York Hospital it was found that 45 patients (10 per cent) had severe or moderately severe personality disturbances, and 90 patients (20 per cent) had relatively mild personality disturbances.

Elsewhere it has been estimated that about 30 per cent of all patients who go to general hospitals and about 50 per cent of all patients seen by general practitioners are

suffering from mental or emotional illness, whether associated with physical illness or not.[7]

The impressive nature of these figures, even granting
their inadequacy as exact statistics, is emphasized by corollary figures relating to so-called "social illnesses." Many
of these, like alcoholism, are to be considered essentially
emotional illnesses, and of others, such as divorce and delinquency, it may be safely said that mental and emotional
illness plays a large role in their causation.

It is estimated that each year 1,750,000 serious crimes are
committed and about 1,500,000 children between the ages
of seven and seventeen are picked up by the police, of whom
about 350,000 are brought to juvenile courts.[8] It is estimated
that there are about 50,000 narcotic addicts and almost
4,000,000 "problem drinkers" in the country at any time.[9]
Of this latter number, about 950,000 are people with severe,
chronic alcoholism. There are about 17,000 suicides each
year and an incalculably greater number of attempts at self-
destruction. For every four marriages there is one divorce.

With all due allowance for the statistical inexactness of
such figures, there can be no doubt that they add up to an
impressive and ominous picture of the distribution of emotional illness in our country. If they err, it is, in my opinion,
on the conservative side; large numbers of instances of the
so-called lesser mental and emotional illnesses are never
recognized as such, and even now the great role such disturbances play in disordered relationships, work dissatis-
factions, absenteeism, accidents of all sorts, marital discord,
and somatic illness is only incompletely recognized. In any
estimate of the seriousness of the situation, we must remember that these statistics do not include the more profound,

and in general less hopeful, mental and emotional illnesses—
the psychoses.

Obviously, no single illness could be responsible for such
a toll of misfortune, and the grouping together of the myriad
and often quite unrelated expressions of emotional dys-
function which are to be discussed here as the neuroses is in
a sense merely a matter of terminological convenience. But
granting that this is so, we must at least attempt a covering,
working definition.

Neurosis is best defined as a maladaptation of the individual in a particular environment at a particular time. It
is always to be looked on as a sickness (disease); it creates
symptoms in the individual which may range from anxiety
to subtle interferences in interpersonal relationships, to inability to experience appropriate emotions, or all the way
to frank interference with such primary functions as eating,
excretion, and sexual performance.

A neurosis results from the interplay of three sets of
forces: (1) the heredity of the individual, (2) his early life
experiences, and (3) the nature of his later life experiences
and difficulties. Psychiatry formerly emphasized hereditary
influences almost to the exclusion of all else. There was a
degree of comfort in this approach, as it absolved the individual from any need to assume much responsibility for the
vagaries of his emotional life, and enabled him to blame
them on his parentage.

Then, later, heredity was almost entirely excluded, and
all the emphasis was placed on the earliest childhood experiences, especially on the relationships between the individual and his parents. The all-important factors influencing
a person's destiny were held to be contained in his earliest
feeding and weaning experiences, habits and modes of toilet

training, and the development of general sexual attitudes, especially the management of the so-called Oedipus situation.

It would be inaccurate and incorrect to imply that psychoanalysis today holds any of these types of experience as less important; rather it may be said that, with greater emphasis on the development of the ego, they are no longer considered as uniquely and selectively important. We realize increasingly (and this recognition was greatly abetted by our experiences during two world wars) that the stress of the life situation plays an immense role in the development of neurotic illness. The experiences of our troops, especially in such situations as Guadalcanal, were of such a devastating nature that large numbers of the best-trained and best adjusted soldiers developed serious emotional difficulties.

A person with poor constitutional equipment may develop a neurosis despite a relatively constructive childhood and in the presence of a life situation not too traumatic in itself. A person may be subject to destructive influences in childhood, and, despite the development of certain neurotic patterns of thought and behavior, find a life situation which is so protective or so undemanding as to enable him to live out a fairly successful life. And life situations other than the excesses of war may tax the defenses of an individual who has previously shown no signs of emotional illness, to the point where clinically significant behavior develops.

In an effort to assay the role of these three sets of factors it is necessary to remember that at least to some degree we are directly responsible for our life situations, and, to complicate matters even more, that our early life experiences may predicate certain choices which will prove overwhelming, such as a bad marriage or an unrewarding and frustrating occupation or career.

Alexander [10] describes a simple and most useful analogy to illustrate this point:

A man buys a truck, and after a while one of its springs breaks. He takes it back to the company saying that the truck broke down because the spring was weak. The company says the truck was all right but that he overloaded it and under such a load it had to break down. Without knowing the quantitative facts precisely this argument cannot be decided. It is obvious that the contention that the spring was too weak is a relative statement—it was too weak for the load. Trucks may break down because of a flaw in construction but a perfectly good truck may also break down under an excessive load.

The only trouble with this, as with all such analogies from mechanical objects to human life, is that it is too static, as though one had excluded any consideration of the heat and humidity to which the truck was subjected, its age, the kind of mechanical care it was given, and similar factors. And for humans, unfortunately, or perhaps fortunately, there will never be "precise quantitative facts"!

Neurotic behavior may be divided into two major groups —the familiar clinically significant types, such as hysteria, compulsive-obsessional neuroses, and the anxiety states, and a larger and equally important group to which less attention has been paid. This is represented by the subtle distortions of ordinary behavior which influence the way we live, work, play, eat, sleep, love, and hate. Although of themselves they may never reach such an intensity as to be clinically significant or cause major disruptions in living, they do influence a wide range of life situations, often with what might be called subclinical but none the less important effects on the productivity and fruitfulness of the individual's life, and of dire consequences in group relations.

I should like now to offer some brief illustrations of both

groups of neurotic manifestations. Of the more familiar
clinical groupings I will make mention of only the anxiety
states, the obsessive-compulsive states, hysteria, and neurotic
character disturbance. This is by no means a complete
list, but should suffice for our purposes.

Anxiety is the symptom par excellence of disturbance
in the emotional life, and it may be part of a whole variety
of clinical entities, often serving as the initial symptom.

Although each of us has on occasion experienced anxiety,
it is extraordinarily difficult to describe. Perhaps the reader's
recollection of how he felt before a crucial examination,
his first big football game, the coming out party, or even the
stroll down the aisle to the altar will do better than words.
The sense of anticipatory dread, unfocused and not quite
localizable; the cold sweaty palms; the palpitation; the urgent and ill-timed call of nature; the tense headache; the
dryness of the mouth—all these are the familiar aspects of
anxiety.

Especially to be noted is the difference between anxiety
and fear. The latter is a necessary, often life-preserving,
reaction to a real danger; if a child did not learn to fear
fire or an oncoming car, he could hardly be expected to
survive. Anxiety is the dread of self-created terror or of a
highly magnified concept or vision of a real object, such
as the dread of a quite harmless pet dog or of insects or
thunder or heights—all objects which derive their capacity
to create anxiety from the individual's symbolization or
projection onto the realistically harmless object. There are
such anxiety elements in the overconcern with health which
endows each pimple with the terror of cancer and makes
each passing headache a symptom of brain tumor. Anxiety
may occur in the presence of certain individuals, in certain

geographic locations, in crowds or at heights, in individuals who seem under other circumstances to be entirely free of any such difficulty.

We may use anxiety to illustrate the general pattern of the development of a neurotic difficulty. The personality is assailed unconsciously by a guilt-producing desire against which the ego [11] must defend itself. The ego must therefore develop defenses by which the anxiety is contained.[12] The clinical form which the neurosis will assume depends in large part on the type of unconscious defense which is employed:

If the causative hostile impulses are turned against the self, depression develops. If they emerge into consciousness as disconnected ideas, an obsessional neurosis may develop. If the hostile impulses are overcompensated by trivial behavior like repeated washing or meticulousness, compulsions result. If they are projected upon others, delusional systems of persecution develop. Sometimes hostile impulses are diffused in general impulsive behavior and in this way a neurotic character disturbance arises. They may periodically overpower the ego as in the manic phase of manic-depressive psychoses. Conversion symptoms may also drain unconscious hostile impulses.[13]

Compulsive-obsessional traits are familiar to most of us from our own experience; as a matter of fact, ritualistic practices are universal in childhood and very common among adults, although of no clinical significance in themselves. Most of us have favorite ways of arranging our desks and our books and making our bedtime preparations, and we are discomfited when changes in these patterns are required. In other words, the need to give up the obsessional pattern produces anxiety by robbing the ego of an established defense. The child's need to take a familiar doll or remnant of a blanket to bed is not very dissimilar to the adult's fussiness about his bedtime reading matter or snack, the arrangement of his pillows, or his favorite sleep-inducing gadget.

From such commonplaces of behavior to clinically significant obsessive-compulsive states is, naturally, a considerable distance. Compulsive acts, such as the familiar hand-washing rituals, compulsive counting, closing of drawers and doors, particular arrangements of objects, are often vast exaggerations of otherwise useful social behavior. These, as well as such profoundly disturbing obsessional ideas as the desire to kill, to have incestuous sexual relationships, to do otherwise repulsive things, are the expression of previously repressed infantile desires.

This type of neurosis strikingly illustrates the struggle between unconscious, repressed desires and tendencies and the repressive force of the ego. The symptoms themselves represent in essence a complex type of unconscious defense against the tremendous anxiety caused by the demands of the forbidden impulses.[14]

Hysteria is a disease long recognized and celebrated in lore and literature. The symptoms which characterize hysteria represent the personality's attempt to express indirectly and in a disguised, symbolic form the repressed unconscious impulses without the intervention of the conscious ego. In fact, hysterical symptoms may be said to have a double symbolic meaning; they express both an unconscious wish and its denial or rejection. The symptoms may range from such interferences with function as result in blindness or paralysis to what is called "the hysterical personality." This is characterized by emotional shallowness and immaturity.

The grosser forms of hysterical manifestations are rare today; it has been years since I saw a (so-called) "grand hysteria" in practice. Instead, we see increasingly the obsessive-compulsive states, character neuroses, and a large number of people who present themselves because of their dissatisfaction with some phase of their life adjustment (work, relationships with people, social usefulness, marital adjustment), for whom an exact clinical diagnosis is often impossible. Wechsler has speculated on this shift as representing a tendency of the neuroses rather to "manifest themselves at higher psychic levels than at the lower physical or somatic levels." [15] I may not agree with this explanation, but I believe the phenomenon he describes is a valid one and an important one for further study.

The so-called character disorders occupy an increasingly important place in psychiatric experience and are seen in ever greater numbers in private practice. It is generally accepted that these patients manifest few of the usual neurotic symptoms (anxiety, phobias, conversion symptoms, and others), but express their neuroses in their general life pattern, in their habitual ways of dealing with life situations, such as work, play, group activity, marriage, and citizen responsibilities. It is difficult to characterize this group in exact terms; they merge with the usual neurotic difficulty on one hand and with the psychopathic personality on the other. These patients are not to be described as weak, wicked, without conscience, or in any other such moralistic terms, but as sick.

The rigid character, the indecisive, the spendthrift, the overemotional person or the one who deals with life by overintellectualizing and by denying feelings, the dominating and the dependent characters, are a few of the familiar disturbances in character. These character manifestations express themselves in behavior unsuited to the individual's life situation (not amenable to the ego's control) and are often productive of great waste and suffering, especially to those with whom the individual lives and works.

In ancient times the emotional and mental ills of people were treated by simple magic, by incantation, by resort to religious practices, by exorcising the reputedly responsible evil spirits, by purges and medicaments supposed to have magical qualities, and so forth.

The quest for proper psychiatric help today is handicapped by lack of knowledge among the great masses of people, the dearth of facilities for treatment, the high cost of obtaining such help, the often lengthy therapy required to accomplish a therapeutic goal, and the host of prejudices and superstitions which still cling to mental and emotional illness and to the fact of being a "psychiatric patient."

The term "psychotherapy" is applied to those psychological methods used to help people with emotional and mental illness. They include a variety of clinical approaches which range from interviews designed essentially to offer the patient reassurance and support, through efforts to manipulate the environment or to help the patient to change a presumably injurious environment all the way to formal psychoanalysis, a highly specialized technique which aims at a basic readjustment in the patient's personality as well as symptomatic relief.

Such a conception of psychotherapy leaves out such procedures as dianoetic healing, the activities of Alcoholics Anonymous, various religious practices which include healing as an essential part of their programs, and other methods.

One can wholeheartedly agree with Knight's statement; "Whoever attempts to evaluate psychotherapeutic methods and practices today finds himself contemplating a modern version of the Tower of Babel." [16] It would be foolhardy,

I believe, and quite unnecessary, to attempt here to bring order from the "confused cries, voices, and languages" of this babel.

Psychotherapy aims variously at increasing the patient's feelings of worth and self-esteem; at affording him an opportunity to gain insight into the nature and motivation of his symptoms and their usefulness in the pattern of his life (his defense systems); at allowing the release of certain hitherto forbidden and repressed impulses under the special circumstances of the therapy; and at increasing his self-acceptance. Always, however, therapy must aim at the alleviation of his difficulties, whether these be in the nature of overt symptoms (anxiety, phobias, somatic dysfunctions, sexual malfunction) or the less clearly defined character disturbances (chronic job failures, inadequate and unrewarding interpersonal relationships, excessive stinginess, and others). Psychotherapy is a term which, as Kubie notes,

> though young, has already acquired too vague and general a meaning. It is used at times for the mystical healing rites of a priest-physician, the drum-beating and the voodoo practices of a modern primitive . . . classes in rhythmic dancing in a modern psychiatric hospital, forced labor in an old prison asylum, the monotone of a class in basket weaving . . . an assortment of modifications of hypnotism or the most subtle and sophisticated psychoanalytic techniques.[17]

Recognizing the claims for such technical innovations as Rogers' "nondirective therapy," hypoanalysis, Moreno's sociodrama, and group therapy, and for the various modifications of the formal psychoanalytic procedures, it can be fairly stated, I believe, that the most useful and satisfactory psychotherapy is that which is based on psychoanalytic theory and awareness and, in suitable cases, psychoanalysis. Certainly I would subscribe to Knight's warning:

I regard the body of knowledge concerning psychopathology and psychodynamics which psychoanalysis has contributed to psychiatry as essential equipment for any doctor attempting major psychotherapy and I feel that the time is long past when this can be considered as a "psychoanalytic bias." In my experience, relatively few patients presenting themselves for psychotherapeutic help are suitable for orthodox techniques, but all of them are entitled to the kind of dynamic assessment and appraisal which psychoanalytic knowledge provides.[18]

Psychoanalysis has as its goal the uncovering and the modifying of unconscious psychological forces, "to broaden the domain of conscious control in human life and to shrink that darker empire in which unconscious forces play a dominant role." [19]

Psychoanalysis requires lengthy treatment (a rough average, of no great statistical accuracy, would be about two to two and a half years, reckoning four or five sessions a week) at considerable cost and utilizing a special technique, based principally on the use of free association. It is a technique whose usefulness in clinically suitable cases is superb; and our knowledge of the conditions for which it is useful increases with the years.

Unfortunately, aside from such important factors as time and expense, there are still far too few analysts, and these are generally grouped in the larger cities. However, psychoanalytically oriented psychotherapy is becoming increasingly available in psychiatric and court clinics, general and psychiatric hospitals, social agencies, and other treatment facilities. Although there is today still a dearth of suitable facilities and trained personnel, the supply of both is steadily increasing, and we have reason to look forward to the ultimate achievement of the goal of therapy available to the emotionally and mentally disturbed in their own communities at reasonable cost. Realistically, we must, however, acknowledge that despite all our best efforts, this is still a long way off.

Of course, the results of the intensive research efforts now under way are unprophesiable, but it is to such research, especially on questions of etiology, that we must look for answers to the problem of the prevention of mental and emotional illness.

3. ADJUSTMENT: ITS USES AND DANGERS

IT IS PERHAPS not unreasonable that after a while a psychiatrist should come to look on the world as one large clinic and its people as so many cases of conflict and disharmony. This is, obviously, a jaundiced perspective, and a psychiatrist must, it seems to me, be careful that his concern with the inner worlds of doubt and anxiety doesn't completely distort his image of those other worlds where adequacy, success and fulfillment are possible.

I am going to discuss, admittedly from a psychiatrist's special perspective, the concept of adjustment and a few of the questions that arise from any consideration of this vast and complicated problem.

Adjustment is a primary need for all people (for all animals, too, for that matter) if they are to survive. The development of the human hand was a superb effort at adjustment; it has been called "the adaptation to end all adaptations." Then there is the process which goes on constantly in the human body to achieve and maintain an effective level of functioning. This process is responsible for a truly amazing array of adaptive changes, many of which go on in the body entirely without the individual's participation or awareness.

Psychologically as well as biologically, beginning at birth, the individual is required constantly to struggle toward an adaptive level which will permit him to survive and to find a suitable place in the society in which he lives: more broadly defined, to be psychologically "well," equating illness for the moment with "maladjustment."

This involves me in some semantic problems, and we had better stop a moment for a few definitions. It is, of course, an oversimplification to speak of mental health as the equivalent of adjustment. But most attempts to define mental health more precisely leave much to be desired.

In the first chapter I have discussed the difficulty of defining emotional adjustment. I have said that perhaps one can describe a well-adjusted person simply as one who holds a job, does not get into trouble with the law, has a reasonably good marriage, enjoys the usual leisure time pursuits commonly available to his group, and is free of anxiety and symptoms which would prevent fulfillment of one's usual round of duties and commitments. If this seems pretty vague and ill-defined I can only assure you it is no more so than many more elaborate efforts; if it seems full of value judgments, I acknowledge this freely and would like to emphasize that it is just this that makes adjustment a fairly tenuous criterion for any estimate of well being.

Adjustment itself has by now become a highly regarded value in our culture, along with happiness, success, fun, mental health, and others. But it is time to ask: who adjusts to what and according to whose standards and values; under what conditions is adjustment a strength and when is it only a pleasant term for the weakness of too easy and uncritical compliance; are all mavericks, crusaders and their unfortunately diminishing like, inevitably to be considered maladjusted and is that *necessarily* something bad and to be avoided?

Marie Jahoda tells of a young man in her native town of Marienthal who found himself at the depth of the depression unemployed and presumably unemployable. Thoroughly discouraged, he decided to take advantage of the fact that in jail the prisoners were offered fairly adequate vocational training. He committed a variety of lesser crimes, found himself in jail, and learned to be an electrician. Armed with his new skill he went to a nearby city and got a job. Jahoda adds, somewhat plaintively, "It is at least a moot question whether his rebellion was mentally not more healthy than the resignation of his elders," [1] a question which neither she nor I can properly answer.

The importance of discussing what we mean by adjustment is underscored by the frequency with which we hear people labeled as "maladjusted," a tag usually meant to imply that such a person is not only "out of step" but neurotic, sick, and a drain on society. This is curiously and unhappily even more common when children, and especially adolescents, are discussed, as if adjustment had become a top value and its absence a sure sign of trouble at hand or ahead. Now, to be sure, with young children especially, certain adjustments or conformities are necessary and need to be learned and adhered to without any ifs, ands, or buts. A child must learn the dangers of fire, exposed heights, oncoming cars, etc., and I always feel free to tell troubled parents who ask me about such situations that they should not hesitate to take matters into their own hands even if it means applying said hand to the seat of Johnny's pants.

But beyond such elementary instances, adjustment must always be thought of in relative terms: in terms of who and when and where and under what circumstances, unless we are willing simply to enshrine conformity and never calculate its dangers to the individual and to society. To settle for conformity is to deny the enormous contributions to our world of the non-conformist, the unusual, the maladjusted. We are grateful for such contributions made throughout recorded history and often revere the memory of those who made them, but we seldom have room in our tight little world for the non-conformists around us, especially those in our own homes.

Perhaps my favorite illustration of the relative nature of adjustment is Eric Hoffer, the author of the highly praised *The True Believer*.[2] His life story is well known, but will bear repeating. In his words, "I had no schooling. I was practically blind up to the age of fifteen. When my eyesight came back, I was seized with an enormous hunger for the printed word." Although no clinical data are available, it is reasonable to assume that his blindness was emotionally induced.

Now middle-aged, Hoffer spent ten years as a migrant worker and since 1943 has worked as a part-time longshoreman. He is determined to remain poor, seeking only to earn enough for his modest daily needs. Entirely self taught, he has now written two interesting and significant books. He lives a tranquil life working for his keep on the docks—an unlikely job for a student—and spending the rest of his time studying and writing—certainly unlikely leisure time pursuits for a longshoreman.

In posing the question of Hoffer's "adjustment," I ask what is perhaps an irrelevant question but one certainly most difficult to answer. To some people his behavior is surely "abnormal," but who is truly privileged to pass such judgment? And if we would agree to call it abnormal, must we not allow that some very fine and creative things may crop up within that category?

I would like to take two further illustrations of this point about adjustment, these from my practice. Some years ago a boy was brought to me because he was failing at school. This boy came from an economically secure home, conservative and eminently correct by every upper-class suburban criterion. The greater, therefore, the parents' horror and dismay when he announced that he wanted to be a "dirt farmer" (which he emphasized when he rejected his father's "gentleman farmer" compromise). This desire to be a farmer, he explained to me, was the reason for his truancy and general misbehavior in school and his surliness and hostility at home. He wanted to flunk; he wanted to get away from the Cadillacs, and the cocktail parties and the horrible questions: how do you like school? Will you be going to Princeton like your dad? Etc., etc.

He was everything his parents were not: simple, unaffected, devotedly loyal to a group of boys of lesser means with whom he shared a love for dogs and bird watching and other seemingly eccentric interests. He truly loved the earth, and found great joy in the unfolding of spring and the new arrival of the flowers and the orderly arrangement of the crops in his vegetable patch. I might add, to illustrate the relative standards by which these things are weighed, that during the war, when this vegetable garden was put in as a patriotic duty, his childish devotion to his assigned chores was called "cute," and he was rewarded as a little patriot. But, so to speak, the war was over . . .

Along about my fifth session with him it suddenly occurred to me (and in retrospect it seems I was woefully slow in understanding) that what purported to be therapy was in essence an effort to get him to accept his family's value system and their way of life. I'll never forget the look of joy on that boy's face when I said I thought he didn't need psychiatric care and that I would talk with his parents about his ambitions. I must say I have rarely had it easier; arrangements were made for him to live with a farm family they knew and go to a country high school. When he graduated he went to an agricultural school in the Middle West, and if messages scribbled on Christmas greetings are any index, I'm sure he's steady on the course to the good life as a farmer.

The second example is that of a college girl of eighteen who consulted me some years ago in a mild but handicapping depression. She was the fourth of five children in a family that made Sanger's Circus seem dull and average. I must not allow myself more than a few recollections of the Joneses; of all the families with whom I have dealt they are perhaps the most vivid. Talented, energetic, enormously endowed physically and mentally, creative, unfettered, they all leapt from achievement to achievement. Everyone painted, read exhaustively, played a musical instrument, fenced, hunted, and swam, wherever possible, in the nude. This last fact will illustrate a part of what I mean. Ann, my patient, never could adjust, not to the nude swimming itself but to its *necessity*, and remembered with bitter tears her humiliation on an occasion when her father teased her unmercifully and accused her of having a middle-class mind. This happened because she refused to swim at all when she first had a young man guest, knowing she would look and be ludicrous in a bathing suit in the midst of all this bounty of nakedness. Her "unusualness" did not end there: she was tone deaf; she chose to attend a traditional girls' college; she joined a sorority; and she became a leader in the Christian Fellowship movement at school. She was actually a quite gifted, warmhearted child. Her maladjustment was more apparent than real and could only be estimated at all as maladjustment if one accepted, as she had, her family's extraordinary standards and behavior as the norm.

I realize, of course, that these are rather extreme examples. Yet I believe that they have the quality and flavor of

the everyday problems and maladjustments of quite ordinary youngsters. Such conflicts frequently arise around
the question of the adolescent's occupational preferences,
where the parents' goals and ambitions so often collide with
a youngster's interests and values. Similarly, old world or
"old hat" ideas about such things as clothes, dating, late
hours, avocational interests, are constant sources of difference, often catalogued as maladjustments. I believe that
we tend to overemphasize these much less extreme forms
of self-expression, and, armed with false values and unreal
expectations, interpret them only too often as clinically significant forms of behavior. In other words, we look on
them as evidences of being "sick."

To be sure, there are many homes where secure parents
accept their youngsters' idiosyncrasies with amused tolerance and even prideful understanding. It is my feeling (and
I admit that I have no statistics to prove this) that this is
less frequent today, that by and large we are not as tolerant
of difference as we once were, and that there is less encouragement for the brave, adventurous living that used to
be considered the American way. And it is likely that we
in psychiatry have contributed to this by constantly pointing out the "meanings" of behavior. We have been more
concerned with suggesting the dangers that lurk in deviations from presumed norms than with emphasizing the
wide range of differences that "normal" rightly must include, or the usually transitory nature of many of these
"abnormal" forms of behavior.

A sensible parent doesn't want his child to adjust *all* the
time; that might make a boy a "sissy," or a girl a nobody,
a wallflower—and what parent wants such a fate for his
children? But on the other hand, and understandably so,
no parent wants his child's rebellion to go so far as to make
him a social outcast, or, even worse, to get him into trouble

at school or with the law. And we seem to have alerted parents to these potential dangers much too thoroughly.

In a sense it is really a matter of values, and values may be subtly manipulated by words. Bertrand Russell has called attention to the possibility of conjugating value-weighted adjectives in such form as:

1. I am firm.
2. You are obstinate.
3. He is a pigheaded fool.

As Felix Cohen pointed out in a brilliant essay, "Almost any human characteristic can be described in honorific or in pejorative terms," and I quote a few of his wonderful illustrations: discreet, cautious, cowardly; loyal, obedient, slavish; kind, soft, mawkish; youthful, young, immature. It depends on who calls the tune and about whom. And it is so easy to be frightened by words. No sensible parent wants his youngster to be a spendthrift but he insists that he be generous; immature is a horror word, young a pleasant and complimentary one; humanitarian laudable, do-gooder derogatory.[3]

Another way to look at this problem is as a struggle between competition and compromise. Competition is instinctive in man; we must learn to compete against the physical environment, against real and symbolic rivals, in school, in business, in romantic conquests—everywhere. As Highet says, "Competition is a natural instinct in the young. Listen to them outshouting and outboasting one another when they are having fun. Watch the innumerable games and stunts which they enjoy, all blended between cooperation and competition, team spirit and rivalry. Think of the more serious competition practiced by adults not only in business and in politics, but in personal display (house, furniture, clothes, cars, and other gadgets), in the craving for publicity and in the innumerable spectator sports on which we spend so many hours and so much money." [4]

It is the control, regulation, and discipline of this competitive need which call for compromise. Either competition or compromise or both in excess can lead to difficulties: the first to a view of life which requires one always to win, always to be better, to do better, to get the other fellow down; the second, to an acceptance of compromise and conformity as guiding principles leading to a readiness to yield on anything to anyone so long as one has "peace and quiet." A good adjustment lies somewhere in between, depending on what may be involved and under what circumstances.

But parents understandably find it difficult to help their children hew to the middle of the road that is considered good adjustment. In the first place, they have been made oversensitive by the well publicized and often contradictory statements of presumed experts and by widely held group mores. Generally speaking, American parents are a little frightened by the image of a child as an "intellectual," especially these days when we live in a climate of heightened anti-intellectualism. Despite all the abundant evidence around us that intellectual achievement is not necessarily an inevitable concomitant of sissiness, parents rather dread it and question the wisdom of such unworldly preoccupations—do the rewards balance the hazards? Naturally this problem of goals and rewards plays an important role in any parent's estimate of the "normalcy" of his youngster; for the father who dreams of his boy as an Ivy League tackle there is small satisfaction in the news that he was elected editor-in-chief of the senior monthly. And, of course, the other way around as well. Even the parent who rejoices in his youngster's intellectual attainments may understandably hope for that leaven of campus success that makes it easier to translate good grades into opportunities for top executive jobs.

Increasingly, parents are apprehensive about adolescent behavior that was once considered typical mischief but is today equated with that dread term juvenile delinquency. The endless scare pieces; the constant exploitation of this theme by politicians with an eye to future elections, by well-meaning reformers of all hues, bringing in their tow psychiatrists and sociologists to "document" their prescriptions—these seem to me to make it almost inevitable that parents will over-react to the sort of transgression which in earlier years would have been passed by without notice, handled with a thrashing or even secretly bragged about.

Now I don't, of course, believe that this is the best of all possible worlds, or that, as almost always happens following great wars and social upheavals, there has not been a considerable increase in so-called delinquent behavior (the "so-called" merely indicates my doubts as to the wisdom of lumping together all sorts of behavioral deviations and labeling them with a term as opprobrious as "delinquent"). And I believe every intelligent step should be taken to study this problem with care and discretion, but in the clinic and in the social laboratory rather than in the scare headlines of the papers. Each of us must recoil with horror at crimes involving youngsters such as those occasional heedless and inscrutable murders, but there is no need to translate them into such immediacy that every parent finds a potential danger in the most insignificant adolescent transgression. A recent newspaper article, written to reassure parents, described six or eight perfectly wonderful American kids; [5]

it was curious to hear it criticized for not selecting "typical" kids, as though the tragic kids from an urban slum were in any sense typical.

What I have been trying to say is embarrassingly simple. I believe we have enshrined, along with other shibboleths of the same kind, the notions of normalcy and adjustment-conformity. At the same time we have apparently failed to reckon the cost both to the individual and to society of this willingness, indeed eagerness, to settle for a lowest-common-denominator estimate of behavior. In the individual such drives for conformity lead to restrictions in human expressiveness and performance. Further, they contribute to the development of hostile, authoritarian approaches to people, and are apt to catalyze prejudice.

We can see the results in the political world today all too clearly. I do not want to compress a highly complicated matter into a sentence or two and risk a misunderstanding. But one needs only to see day by day the retribution visited on individuals for the slightest deviation from a political norm imposed in the name of security, but inflicted by rigid conformists terrified by the merest shadow of deviation. As Learned Hand has expressed so beautifully in his brilliant essay on liberty, "My thesis is that any organization of society which represses free and spontaneous meddling is on the decline, however showy its immediate spoils; I maintain that in such a society liberty is gone, little as its members know it; that the Nirvana of the individual is too high a price for a collective paradise . . . our collective fate in the end depends upon the irrepressible fertility of the individual and the finality of what he chooses to call good." [6]

Although I have not tried to offer a remedy and could not even if I had space, I should like only to suggest to parents and others that we try to take it easy in our application of complicated psychological-ethical standards to living people, especially youngsters. I should like to believe that patience, sympathy, love, understanding, and, for that matter, time itself, will help resolve many a problem; and to remind you that our country began and grew strong in the beliefs and actions of non-conformist individuals who were not afraid.

4. ADOLESCENCE

ALL OF US were once adolescents. If adults could really remember that simple truth, we would automatically advance in our understanding, and probably in our management of the usual adolescent problems.

Like other such pieces of advice, that dictum is not quite so simple as it seems. Adolescence is a period of turbulent self-questioning and struggle for everyone, and a time of great humiliation and shame and of a deep feeling of inadequacy for many. That is why we tend to repress our memory of the experience, to try to forget about it. Certainly, we adults would like to believe that we were never the querulous, demanding, unpredictable, sulking, unappreciative characters that those adolescents with whom we must now deal almost always are. All the clichés about the younger generation reflect the success with which adults have managed to forget, to deny what their own adolescence was like. With this in mind I have tried to derive from my experience with young people some general conclusions about adolescence, with only a passing reference to those deviations that are so striking and serious.

The problems of adolescent delinquency and of those profoundly disturbing neurotic conflicts which have such extreme reverberations in family and school situations have been more or less adequately dealt with in psychiatric and lay literature. A really disturbed adolescent can create havoc in a household. The hostility of such a youngster may provoke the adults in his environment from tolerance and patient forbearance to a retaliatory show of strength and often to overt hostility. And this establishes a vicious cycle that ultimately involves the child, his brothers and sisters, parents, grandparents, friends, teachers—in short, everyone with whom he is in contact—in a frenzy of trying to deal adequately with the consequences of his behavior. Such situations are beyond easy understanding and eventually require some kind of treatment.

I prefer to discuss adolescence as the inevitable period between childhood and adulthood, a time of rapid physical, mental, and emotional change as well as of basic choice-making.

The biological, emotional, and intellectual growth which ordinarily accompanies adolescence, which in a real sense *is* adolescence, confronts the youngster with a whole array of problems. And, although it seems trite and obvious, they descend on him before he is at all ready for them. To this fact the adults' recurrent theme, "If I could only do it over again, knowing what I know now," pays eloquent testimony. The biological, emotional, and intellectual changes are tremendous—how tremendous we do not usually stop to recall. The crack in the adolescent boy's voice, the ungainly mannerisms, the pudgy obesity seem pretty funny to adults. But to the youngster they are sources of painful embarrassment and, more significantly, they are the outward signs of a physical and psychological revolution. This involves, of course, the complicated process of sexual maturation and all the physical and emotional changes that necessarily accompany it. The younger child yearns to grow up, to be like an adult. The growing girl anticipates menstruation, and her male counterpart practices shaving a nonexistent beard.

But with adolescence it is as though such fooling around with being a grownup comes to a halt and the youngster must get down to the business of maturing. He has been evicted from childhood, and the loss of its protection and the vista of adulthood with all its responsibilities seem utterly appalling. As long as he could cling to the privileges of childhood he was not quite so frightened at the prospect of being an adult. But now adolescence forces him to recognize that adulthood is near at hand, and all the successive physical changes serve as constant reminders. As if this weren't enough, his elders frequently put it into words for him: "You're not a child any more."

The adolescent caught in this twilight zone, no longer a child but not yet an adult, turns increasingly to his peers and to those slightly older for approval and understanding. He can no longer share "kid stuff"; he is suspicious and wary of adults; his own gang offers him solidarity, interest, and the common bond of shared doubts and hostilities. It is partly to this need that the formation of destructive adolescent gangs may be attributed. On the other hand, this impulse to group cohesion, properly directed and nurtured, can stimulate most useful and healthy group activities. Clubs, teams, and other associations often afford important testing grounds for interests and talents. Not infrequently membership in them is the beginning of important lifelong friendships and activities.

At the same time, this group identification also accounts for many of the excesses that make adolescent behavior so troublesome and often so sad. Keeping up with the gang often leads the youngster to behavior that he would have had neither the desire nor the courage to initiate on his own. In the group, bluster and bluff are necessary; at home they make the adolescent a little grotesque and pathetic.

In my experience I have often noted that much of the adult's impatience and displeasure result from this inappropriateness of adolescent behavior, its fumbling inadequacy and its futility. An average parent probably would not mind it so much if only the youngster were not seemingly so cocky about his doings, and so clearly frightened at the same time, and so helpless when confronted by rejection and failure.

The truculence of the adolescent boy's behavior is influenced in good part by two important cultural phenomena. In the average American family the father is out of the home practically all day and has little time to spend with his children. Although the shorter work day and week have done a good deal to change this, and there are gratifying changes in the attitudes of many fathers, especially younger ones, it may still be said that the American youngster is subject to predominantly feminine influences. And this is true not only of the home but also of the school, where the great majority of teachers in the early school years are women.

In the effort to free himself from such powerful feminizing influences, the adolescent boy assumes the attitudes of a compulsive, aggressive masculinity and strives, prematurely and clumsily, to assert what he thinks are masculine prerogatives and to revolt from the standards and practices of the home which he considers feminine. Naturally, as is true of all such revolutions, this one, too, is given to excesses. Now nothing the boy has learned at home is any longer to be considered good, and the specter of being a sissy hounds him to rebellion and disobedience. This ranges from the relatively innocent physical sloppiness to drinking, smoking, swearing excesses, and their companion, sexual braggadocio. (True, sloppiness is no longer solely a masculine prerogative. I wonder when the male adolescent, viewing the girl's self-conscious, imitative sloppiness in dress and manner, will give it up as no longer a useful protest against being a sissy!) The revolt from femininity is also involved in the group cohesion of which I spoke above, and is often responsible for some of the less healthy aspects of group activity.

The problem of the adolescent girl is not so clearly understood and is greatly complicated by the physical changes of adolescence in the female. In general, adults seem to be more tolerant of the excesses and idiosyncracies of the adolescent girl. Traditionally, adolescent girls are thought of as weaker and more delicate than their brothers. The beginning of the menstrual cycle usually elicits a greater degree of patience than does the biological development of boys. However, it would seem that the "clinging-vine" adolescent girl is pretty much out of style for the moment and the tomboy in the ascendancy, with the current "uniform" of turned-up blue denims and a man's shirt (tails out) everywhere to be seen. Nor are the gang aspects so familiar among girls, although the same drive is present in the cliques and clubs favored by them. Just what cultural changes, of which such shifts in dress and attitudes are an indication, will result cannot be seen; nor is it plain what, if any, basic change may result in the community's attitude toward the adolescent girl, or, for that matter, in her attitudes toward herself and her world.

We are all familiar with the usual adolescent crush on a camp counselor, a teacher, a somewhat older schoolmate, or, for that matter, on a national hero figure of the same sex. These crushes are an expression of the homosexual component that is a part of the sexual life of all human beings, and is in fact the expression of perfectly normal sexual interests. The intensity of such crushes often causes parents considerable concern. This is especially true when the adolescent is so absorbed in the relationship that more usual social contacts are excluded; and particularly when the crush is associated with some form of overt sexual behavior, even though this is slight and incomplete.

To discuss this phase of sexual maturity in any detail is beyond the scope of these remarks. I think it can be regarded as part of the choice process that confronts everybody at adolescence. Obviously the vast majority of people "choose" heterosexuality and find satisfaction for their homosexual impulses in the socially acceptable outlets of friendship and the like. Of course it must be emphasized that this is in no sense a conscious choice; it is to be understood as a phase of the individual's entire life story.

An important part of the solution of this sexual problem is the handling of the youngster's attachment to his parents, especially the parent of the opposite sex. A healthy solution depends in good measure on the degree to which the child has been enabled to form healthy dependencies. This means that the dependencies must not be so excessive as to demand their prolongation into adulthood or so exclusive as to make painful, if not impossible, the shift to another adult love object. This sort of useful environment will allow healthy relations with brothers and sisters which will inevitably include an opportunity for the child to become aware of hostility and jealousies (especially as between boy and girl) and to be allowed a reasonable degree of freedom in verbal and other expression of such feelings. In a sense, the child first confronts our competitive society within his own family situation and must really learn there—if he is ever to learn—the give-and-take and the respect for other

people's needs and rights which are so necessary for successful living.

In our culture, the accepted method of heterosexual experimentation is dating and its concomitants, necking and
petting. The adolescent's almost religious need to define
precisely the difference between these two is good evidence of the kernel of his dilemma: He wants to be like his
elders, which (he thinks) requires fairly venturesome sexual experimentation; but he needs to maintain the esteem of
his own group, which actually condemns too daring sex-
uality, even when seeming to approve it.

I remember a patient, a young college freshman, torn
by the wish to be like the upperclassmen and "know
women," but afraid to be different from his friends who
did not venture anything more than the innocuous necking
he himself had already experienced. He had the questionable
luck to meet a girl who, though his own age, had indeed
had extensive heterosexual experience. He fled in panic
both from her excessive demands and easy availability and
from his awareness that his closest friends resented his boast-
ing which seemed to belittle their relatively puny successes.
He found his solution in a self-righteous morality that con-
demned the girl's promiscuity and allowed him safety from
her sexual demands. In addition, this attitude afforded him
a smug satisfaction in the moral superiority of his behavior
and facilitated a quiet return to the dating routine accepted
by his group.

Adolescence is the time of another important choice—
the choice of one's lifework. With few exceptions, this too
is a final choice; once they have decided on a field of work,
few people have the opportunity to change it. Where education and training are basically involved, few can afford
the luxury of re-education and retraining. Even when ex-

pense is not a consideration, a choice commits one to a whole way of life, often to a geographical location, and it is rarely that one can undo such decisions once they have been made.

The finality of the decision, once made, is only one of the reasons why the choice of an occupation is of such great importance. In ordinary human values, the satisfactions and contentment an individual derives from his job must obviously stand very high indeed. In fact, job dissatisfaction is one of the greatest and most pressing social problems; among the causes of such discontent an unsuitable occupational choice is an important one.

Quite early in life the child may seem to be concerned with what he wants to be. Adults' questions seem to be restricted to the trilogy: "What class are you in?" "Do you like school?" "What do you want to be?" For the very young child the answer to the last question is, of course, sheer fantasy; a little boy wants to be like a grownup and hence like Pop or some current hero.

It is only as the growing youngster begins to discover his interests and to test them against his capacities and skills that the task of making an occupational choice begins to take form. As adolescence advances, an important and often decisive new element is added; the youngster is increasingly concerned with the values of contemplated jobs. "To work with people" seems an important reason for going into personnel work, for instance, or "to help people" a good one for choosing medicine as a career. The simple identification processes so clearly present in earlier choices, are, if active at all, made to conform to the compelling factors of interests, skills, and values.

This is a process that reaches a peak during the late adolescent years. Children of the more economically secure, who will probably go on to college, face successive choices, such as the college to attend, what to major in, and whether to plan on graduate work or to terminate formal education with college. For the youngster whose education must end with high school (or before) problems of possible vocational training, civil service jobs, and other decisions require definition and decision in these years.

Aside from the immediate importance of these choices, they have corollaries of great consequence. The poorer boy who leaves high school in the second year abandons almost all ambition for further intellectual advancement or even rigorous mechanical training. Hence he is free to devote much of his time to leisure pursuits, including, of course, sexual ones. The boy who has a set of life plans that include years of study and training must forego this immediate satisfaction, postponing today's gratifications for tomorrow's good. This must reflect a whole hierarchy of values which will enable him to forego direct sexual satisfaction for the more subtle gains that contribute to the working out of a suitable occupational choice.

In general, occupational choice seems to be a much less pressing problem for girls, even for those who plan to work. This reflects the quiet certainty with which the girl recognizes marriage as her first and inevitable goal. The problem then is for her to attain that goal and reconcile within it some expression of a talent, an interest, or a skill, perhaps by way of avocational pursuits.

A third and compelling problem demands the concern of parents and educators: the problem of religious expression and affiliation. Understandably, at this time in history, this is a more immediate problem for certain religious groups. But it has some urgency, if a lesser one, for all adolescents. They are as a group, after all, quite disillusioned about everything, especially the things grownups do and believe, and this includes religious beliefs and practices. It is in the field of religious activity that one often finds most clearly revealed still another adolescent characteristic. To the youngster the world is a great and wide-flung challenge, and he is about to rescue it from the evils for which those incompetents, his elders, are responsible. Nothing seems too remote or too difficult. A startling shift to orthodoxy may represent this new attitude toward religion, and here, too, one finds a trying smugness and complacency and a high degree of intolerance for the beliefs and practices of adults. The specific working out of this problem varies from family to family; it is never solved, any more than any other adolescent problem, by a show of force or authority.

To understand adolescents it is important to remember that they are bewildered, frightened, and confused. An adolescent patient of mine did a series of beautiful and expressive surrealistic paintings to express her feelings; woven in the design of one of them is the phrase, "I'm a stranger here myself." I could think of no expression truer or more revealing. The adolescent finds his newly approaching adulthood strange indeed; he finds the departure from childhood frightening, and the attitude and the demands of the adult world little short of terrifying.

To help them, adults must understand them. Young people welcome the expressed recognition by adults, especially parents, that they too once were adolescents and behaved in pretty much the same way. Although suspicious and distrustful of the grownups' motives, boys and girls will profit by good-humored explanations especially when an adult is not aloof.

What makes the situation difficult for the parent, though, is the fact that love, generosity, kindness, permissiveness are often not enough to deal with the adolescent's problems.

After all my years of experience, in fact, I know of nothing that so completely defied any generalized prescription as adolescence. I believe this is so because its conditioning begins in the cradle. I often feel that in the end the only solace for adolescent and adult alike is the recognition that this too passes.

5. VALUES AND THE PSYCHIATRIST

THE PROBLEM of values is an ancient one; when the people of Israel were admonished that the Lord did not ask of them "burnt offerings and the calves of a year old" and that He would not be pleased with "thousands of rams or with ten thousands of rivers of oil" but that He had shown what was required, namely, "to do justly and to love mercy and to walk humbly with thy God," [1] man was confronted with problems which in their modern dress are those of value.

A value is a criterion which helps us to distinguish between alternatives and affords us a base for recognizing ourselves in relation to the rest of the world.

Such a choice between alternatives, which is the essence of the problem of values, is clearly made in Micah's plea to his people; indeed, throughout the entire history of the Western world, rich in its Judaeo-Christian tradition, such problems have been ever present. Aristotle held that value qualities were supreme over all the other attributes of things and Plato called the problem of values the most difficult of all science. Great names in the history of human thought have struggled with the problem of values: Kant, Nietzsche, Adam Smith, Marx, Ricardo, Dewey, and others. And

American philosophy for two decades has been preoccupied with the theory of value.

But it is not only the professional student of philosophy who has been so greatly concerned; recently it seems the word "value" and the concepts of "value systems," "value judgment," "hierarchy of values," etc., have gained a quite extraordinary place in our everyday speech and writing. Again and again I am surprised when patients use these terms in the quite ordinary currency of speech, patients of whom one would not anticipate such usage either from their education or any discernible preoccupation with philosophical matters. In the press, in fiction, in the theater, in scientific essays originating from a host of varied disciplines, one finds values discussed; from the "values" of the market place to those of the "good and the beautiful," there is a quite obvious concern with this problem.

It may be that I am projecting my own concern with these questions of value and hence overemphasizing the presumed preoccupation which people have with this problem, but the notion of this widespread interest in value problems persists and I do not think the phenomenon, if I assay it correctly, is difficult to explain. We live in a time of extraordinary tension and have only now passed through, or, perhaps better, are still passing through, a crucial period in history. Is it not natural that we are confronted with the need for a critical moral re-evaluation of our civilization and of our role within it? And since the problems of values lie at the very core of our mores and our beliefs, it seems only natural that the word and the concept should have come into more or less everyday usage. In periods of rapid change and frightening challenges to society's very existence, all men are confronted with the necessity for resolving conflicts resulting from the fact that their old values cannot cope with the new reality.

But despite the centuries-long study of the complicated problems of values and despite the contributions of philosophers, economists, and social scientists, psychiatry and psychoanalysis have had surprisingly little to say on the subject, though it seems to me obviously at the very heart of our work and, as with other individuals, of our lives. This chapter will try to deal with the role of value systems in the psychoanalytically oriented psychiatrist's life and work. Although some of my comments apply directly to psychoanalysis and psychoanalysts, I believe that what I shall have to say applies in essence to all of us who work with people: psychiatrists, psychologists, social workers, social psychologists, etc. Partly because of the limitations of space but also because I am not a philosopher or anything more than an amateur student of ethics and morals, I shall not attempt any detailed consideration of such involved and frequently obscure problems as the relation of values to morals, the role of the will in human behavior, the relation of values to language and symbols, etc. I have the more modest goal of discussing certain relatively simple problems of values as they are found in our everyday jobs and in our everyday lives, without too much concern—at least in this place—with a systematic analysis of the value problem.

According to Robin Williams, values may be defined as "affectively charged conceptual structures registered by the individual which act as directives. They form an important part of the apprehension of self and act as directional factors in the organization of behavior." [2] In perhaps more simple terms, values are essential parts of our self-regulating system, reflecting our needs, standards, interests and goals, and are inevitably tested in specific life situations. They are influenced by our feelings of shame and guilt and measured by our reactions of self-appreciation. Values not only reflect our inner needs and our personal system of choices, but they are clearly influenced by the cultural system and its sanctions and disapprovals. In other words, while a value must satisfy one's own inner standards, it must also meet with the approval of the group as a whole or at least be in harmony with the standards of a large subgroup.

In more explicit psychoanalytic terms, value judgment is not a purely conscious, intellectual process but reflects as well unconscious processes whereby the instinctual demands of the individual, the superego requirements and the needs of the ego are successfully or otherwise expressed in an individual's attitudes. In general, such psychoanalytic writings as there are on the subject of values stress the superego factors, really equating values with morals (as in Sommers,[3] Flugel,[4] etc.).

To some extent an exception to this statement is found in Fromm's [5] work, in which values are equated largely with ethics and the ego aspects given considerable prominence. I, too, would rather view the problem as essentially a problem of ego psychology; and while this does not in any way minimize the role or importance of unconscious determinants, I believe that a proper understanding of values must emphasize the functioning of the ego directed toward the world of reality, the world of ultimate adjustment and behavior. Important aspects of ego function are reflected in our values: the question of interests and goals, the problem of the postponability of satisfactions, and the acceptance of compromise solutions of our instinctual demands are a few. We develop our value systems much as we develop our other character traits: through the influences of early life experiences, especially the nature and strength of our identification with key figures in our childhood.

All of us constantly need to revise our values in terms of their tension-producing or easing qualities, their influence in adaptation and their role in the reality situation. It is essential to remember that our values are not static but require evaluation and modification throughout our lives; without such capacity to deal with values, there would be little social growth or progress. Values are often used to maintain the *status quo;* they are likewise instrumental in developing social change.

To turn quite abruptly from this introduction, I should like to discuss the relation of values to psychiatry under these general headings: value judgments and the occupational choice of the psychiatrist; value judgments in the choice of patients and in their treatment, including some comments on the termination of treatment; and, finally, the social role of the psychiatrist.

In general, the problem of work is one replete with important value considerations. In a study [6] of the determinants of occupational choice, my colleagues and I have emphasized the significant role played by value judgments in this choice process. We found, for example, that youngsters of eleven expressed values when they said they wanted to work "where they could help people," an idea, incidentally, which was frequently advanced as a basic consideration as to why they wanted to become doctors or nurses. Young adolescents of twelve to fourteen recognize the values that they hope to realize through work—"to work for a good life"; "to work outdoors" or "to work where one can travel" or "to have an exciting job," "a well-paid job," etc. However, it is a bit later, at sixteen or so, that values emerge as focal centers in the occupational choice pattern. By this time genuine interests have begun to crystallize, unsuitable choices have been relinquished, capacities tested, opportunities explored and, finally, there emerges a value system tempered to fit all these considerations.

Although obviously psychiatrists too have made an occupational choice in which their own value systems must have played a determining role, one finds that little or nothing has been written concerning this. At one time or another during our study of occupational choice, I asked a dozen or so colleagues, in an entirely informal way, why they thought they had become psychoanalysts. Had I not had previous experience on a more extensive and formal basis of inquiring of psychoanalysts concerning the determinants of occupational choice in certain of their analysands, I would have perhaps been more amazed than I was. Certainly the role of their own value judgments was not conspicuously important to any of them (with a single exception). In general, their explanations followed the familiar analytic concept of the occupational choice problem and represented various types of transformations of instinctual drives and identification processes. I do not want to repeat here our already published conclusions about the inadequacy of these explanations for any occupational choice; we do not believe that such factors by any means represent an adequate explanation though they certainly are of significant importance in contributing to the choice.

But what I derived from these chats with my colleagues was a feeling that we are almost ashamed or afraid to examine our own values, almost like the youngster who similarly denies such values as "humanitarianism" or "idealism" for fear that he may be considered a "sissy."

Even the commonplace value of earning a good living was denied or apologized for. Freud said without hesitation: "Anyone who wanted to make a living from the treatment of nervous patients must clearly be able to do something for them." [7]

This failure to be willing to face the problem of money in our work leads to such questionable economics as are revealed in a recent book on psychoanalysis which states:

"Perhaps it is relevant to add that the psychoanalyst contributes working capital to every treatment, in that he gives his patients his only irreplaceable goods, *Time*. [Author's italics.] The hours which he devotes to his patients are his only working capital; and what he expends on one patient cannot be used for another." [8] I need hardly point out that this is as true of any other professional person, or for that matter, of every carpenter or toolmaker; what concerns me more is this need for apology and rationalization which grows out of our feelings that money is a base value and that earning it must be somehow explained away and excused.

Sachs,[9] in one of the few published contributions concerning analytic training, says: "To enter a profession because one wants to make a living and hopes to make a living by it, is a perfectly honest and legitimate endeavor. All that is asked is a thorough training, conscientious work, industry and integrity. That earning money [10] is a leading motive in the choice of a profession is no reason for withholding training *except in psychoanalysis*. [My italics.] This is a point of difference which springs from the fundamental fact that psychoanalysis is not just another medical specialty, not simply a branch of psychiatry but emphatically *a res generis*. . . . Psychoanalysis demands all of a man's humanity."

This statement of Sachs clearly is a statement of his own value judgments and however much shared by any of us, and hence admired, cannot be otherwise considered. It happens that at this time psychiatry and psychoanalysis are ways to earn a good living, and while I should not like to appear a crass materialist, I think the denial represents a false value goal.

Why must there inevitably be a clash between "a man's humanity" and earning a good living? There are certainly other than the "merchandising" values in our work; this whole consideration is part of the larger problem of rewards and goals. For instance, such conflicts in values are basic in the choice between full-time institutional work and private practice; they vitally influence the entire problem of obtaining adequate training and especially psychoanalytic training.

Furthermore, I believe such questions of value are of greater importance in the clash between various schools of thought in our work than is acknowledged, for instance, in the continuing struggle about psychologists as psychotherapists. Matters of prestige and especially of earning power are values which play an important role in this conflict; I do not recall ever having seen this freely acknowledged in discussions concerning it.

Another problem of values which is an important and constant part of the therapist's life and work reflects a similar set of concerns: Whom, in a world where only a fraction of those who need it can be treated, is the analyst to treat? Naturally there are the clinical considerations which are and always must be given first importance in eliminating those completely unsuitable for treatment. But are there not other considerations of perhaps secondary but still great importance? The clash between the realities of harsh economics and the need to choose our patients, at least in good part, on the basis of fees is often unpleasant and distasteful indeed, but needs to be faced much more frankly and considered not only in terms of the patients but also in terms of the conditions of work it imposes on us. I do not mean to suggest that this is uniquely a problem faced by psychoanalysts (though obviously the circumstances and conditions of our work set our job somewhat apart) or to hint at some special lack in ourselves that makes us peculiarly vulnerable to such considerations. For a discipline with such ambitious goals as ours and a therapy and training in such short supply, these are problems that cannot be avoided or relegated to oblivion by ignoring them. We have all had the wonderful experience of treating, perhaps for a "token" fee, a fine scientist or creative person early in his career and then, perhaps years later, learning of an important scientific or artistic contribution made by such a person. Analysts are not above satisfactions of the vicariously shared "triumph," and we need to examine the inevitable conflict that our own value schemes impose when we work in a world of harsh choices and painful compromises. I think this problem is especially acute to those of us who work in or on the periphery of a university, where financial rewards are at best modest and the demands on us to help young academicians a constant problem in our work lives.

Perhaps you will be glad to have me put aside such mundane matters as fees and the limitation of our time and energies as against the demands made upon us. I admit I do it gladly. But value judgments are important in many other aspects of our therapeutic work and their consequences not always fully acknowledged. So much of our work is necessarily directed to the understanding of the unconscious forces in the patient that even in our insights into ego problems we are largely concerned with the unconscious elements. In addition, we still seek what I believe is a spurious goal in our quest for objectivity; what we need is a recognized subjectivity, a free and acknowledged awareness of our own values and the role they play in our therapeutic efforts. *The analyst, too, has values and must face them.* This requires not only that he recognize his own values, but that he examine the social realities about him and his own position in the cultural scheme and the demands placed upon him in terms of his own values. I have often thought that our claim that we have no blueprint

for our patient, that we want him only to be free to transform his instinctual needs into meaningful and healthy patterns of living, is illusory. Analysts must work with a definition of what constitutes the mental and emotional health
they are trying to enable the patient to achieve; that such a
definition must reflect the analyst's own values seems self-
evident.[11]

To take a simple example of what I mean: A patient
brought up in a family close to the end of its financial pre-
eminence but still clinging desperately to symbols of prestige, social stratification, the formalities of social intercourse,
etc., enters treatment. I took almost for granted that part of
the therapeutic goal would entail a shift in this patient's
value system as well as an understanding of the unconscious
dynamic forces involved in her illness, and that this new
value system would inevitably reflect my own (or any other
therapist's to whom she might have gone), modified, of
course, in the complexities of the transference situation.
For her, to take a job (and a simple, ill-paid one at that,
for she lacked completely any training or skills that would
have prepared her to earn a living); to move her residence
to independent, but extremely modest, quarters; to find
friends among outgroups she had previously despised; to
travel by subway and bus; to eat lunch in a cafeteria, a
symbol of all she had previously despised as "beneath her";
were all as important as understanding her unresolved attachment to her uncle (her main "father" figure). Indeed,
they clearly went together and represented two aspects of
the same process. I am not sure if in this case her values could
have been altered outside the therapeutic situation, though
it is well known that decisive, positive life experiences outside of treatment frequently do permit such shifts in values.
(By way of parenthesis, this is brilliantly exemplified in the
life stories of many Europeans who were compelled to flee

from their homes. I have seen time and time again the unbelievable shifts in values many of these people were able to make and the satisfying life adjustments which have resulted.) Therapy enabled my patient to relax her rigid superego, a necessary precursor to her acquisition of a new value system, and gave her a set of values she could live up to, a prerequisite to any reasonably healthy adjustment.

I remember vividly a "spoiled darling of the rich" I had seen a dozen or so times in treatment only to have her discontinue with an utterly condescending and impudent letter. I was to learn only years later that she had fallen in love with a young scientist who told her bluntly that if she wanted to marry him she would have to disavow her entire way of life. When she returned seeking help for a difficult personal problem, she was in almost every way unrecognizable. She had, through the strength of her love relationship with her strong and emotionally healthy husband, been enabled to effect a complete shift in her values. Or, I might speculate on the extraordinary shift in values so frankly and courageously related in Mrs. Roosevelt's fascinating autobiography.

Among the most important ego functions is the capacity to postpone instinctual gratifications. The role of the value hierarchy is clearly basic in the development of this ability. A choice which enables one to persevere at a difficult or dull task rather than to forego it for some immediate libidinal pleasure must inevitably entail a recognition and acceptance of the satisfactions of the completed task, a meaning which in turn must encompass the value attached to the task performed in contrast to the self-denied pleasure.

In recent investigations of such matters as prejudice, political deviations, occupational choice, etc., a curious lack in what the analyst hears (so to speak) has come to our attention and represents, I believe, another aspect of a value problem. For instance, numbers of analysts when asked about anti-Semitism in their analysands stated that they had not even encountered the problem. I believe it is impossible to explain this on technical grounds, such as the failure of the prejudice to play an important role in the therapeutic situation, and that it probably represents the analyst's own value system which keeps him from ascribing any real importance to the problem of prejudice. Similarly I do not believe that the relative barrenness of psychoanalytic investigation into the question of the choice of occupation represents only, or even largely, the limitations imposed by the therapeutic situation, but rather a sort of selection imposed unconsciously by value concepts. Certainly for an analyst who believed, let us say, that the nature of a man's work was unimportant unless it created neurotic problems, questions of occupational choice would seem relatively secondary. The instinctual aspects of the problem are, as usual, well understood but the reality-directed aspects barely touched upon.

In the use of psychoanalysis as a research device, yet another value problem is of major concern. An earlier extreme attitude permitted such a comment as ". . . There is the subjective difficulty of maintaining scientific detachment in the study of human affairs. Few human beings can calmly and with equal fairness consider both sides of a question such as socialism, free love or birth control. Opinions on these matters are not viewed with the ethical maturity with which we view opinions as to the structure of protoplasm, the ether, the atom, etc." [12] (Parenthetically, we must remark on the naïveté which led Professor Cohen, the author of these remarks, to include the atom as a subject we view with "ethical maturity," although, naturally, he could hardly have anticipated the bomb. We shall want to return to the atom a bit later!) Here clearly stated is the notion of the

sanctity of objectivity, an unawareness that in every step of
social research conscious and unconscious value judgments
play a decisive role. As Myrdal has said, "There is no other
device for excluding biases in social sciences than to face
the valuations and to introduce them as explicitly stated,
specific premises." [13] "Without valuations," says Professor
Wirth, "we have no interest, no sense of relevance or of significance and consequently no object." [14] It has been said
that the reason social scientists do not more often arrive at
the truth is that they frequently do not want to. And often
values themselves are utilized as resistance to social change.
The desire to attain the truth is, after all, a late and relatively
undeveloped human motive compared with the more vital
motives of social approval. I wonder how much the relative
lateness of psychoanalytic concern with ego problems as
against the problems of instinctual (id) energies reflects the
difficulties which are immediately encountered in all such
inquiries.

Even the problem of termination in therapy, for which
we have few highly accurate or satisfactory criteria, will
reflect in part the analyst's concept of the world, his own
and the patient's, and hence mirror his own value scheme.
It is obvious that no complete resolution of conflict is ever
possible (remember Freud's warning that psychoanalysis
could only restore patients to health and to "everyday unhappiness"). An important aspect of the decision as to what
constitutes "tolerable conflict" in a given individual will require some estimate of a person's social usefulness and social
contribution, and this in turn will reflect the therapist's
own values. An analyst to whom I had referred a young
woman expressed considerable dissatisfaction with the conclusion of the analysis because the patient still attended
church. Though I cannot at this time discuss at length my
viewpoint on the question of religion and mental health,

I might say that in this instance discussion with my colleague clearly revealed that what was disturbing him was his own value system, which allowed no room at all for religious observance and overlooked entirely the patient's surely equally valid set of values of which her religious practices were an important part.

Another patient who had come to treatment because of episodes of mild but debilitating depression was encouraged to interrupt her treatment, to return to college and then prepare for a career in a science for which she had special and rather rare native capacities. She had for the ten or more years of her marriage led an exceptionally barren existence, which was nominally distasteful to her but to which she thought herself chained by the handicaps imposed by her fits of depression. To be sure, her therapeutic work enabled her to confront the problem and tackle it; the resulting shift in her values and in her reality situation not only enriched the therapy but gave her quite literally a new sense of the value of her life.

Much of this is commonplace in our work; every choice a patient makes—a job, a spouse, an avowed cause, an assumed obligation—has values involved in it, and much of the work of the therapist will reflect his insight into these values. It is necessary, I believe, for the development of our own science that such concern with values should be acknowledged and its implications for the therapeutic process systematically explored.

The analyst must deal not only with the inner compliance of the patient but also with compliance to the social norms represented in an accepted value system. For instance, a patient terminated her analysis with me by mutual agreement. Some years later she saw the need for further help and sought this in another city to which she had moved. In discussing her situation the colleague to whom I had referred her commented: "Almost the first thing that struck me about Mrs. X was her insistence on employing Negro domestics and her overcompensatory [his word] interest in them and Negroes in general." The patient and I had worked extensively with this; in part, it reflected her early childhood experiences with a traditional "mammy," and in part her unconscious overevaluation of the Negro as a sexual object. The dynamics of this particular bit of behavior are not our concern at this time; what I should like to emphasize is my colleague's immediate rejection of such attitudes as incompatible with good mental health, to my mind clearly a reflection of his own value scheme.

Which properly brings me to the last facet of this problem. In a recent essay on ethical science, Professor Morgenau of Yale says: "What matters today is not whether ideas on ethics are original but whether they work in our world." [15] I do not know if I have any ideas that will "work"; I should like to sketch my concept of the social role of the psychiatrist, hoping that it may suggest an approach to a program which may "work."

Elsewhere [16] I have written of a meeting with a group of young atomic scientists which I think was the first occasion I had to become truly aware of the deep need for each of us to re-examine his role in society and the value systems reflected in this role. Here were a group of devoted scientists, in branches of science traditionally considered "pure" [17] and hence outside the realm of ethics and teleology, who had in fact suspended their active scientific work to propagandize on the ethical meaning of atomic energy and its future use. Since then I have read much that atomic scientists have written; what soul searching and what a shattering awareness of the social implications of their work! If indeed values are tested by us in terms of their guilt- and shame-producing capacities, here are people struggling with a value problem as keenly as if they had personally solved the riddle of fission or, for that matter, had released the bomb over Hiroshima. J. Robert Oppenheimer, in discussing his reaction to the explosion of the first atom bomb on July 16, 1945, observed, "In some crude sense which no vulgarity, no humor, no over-statement can quite extinguish, the physicists have known sin; and this is a knowledge which they cannot lose."

We as psychiatrists also need to examine our own social role, even though luckily our awareness of guilt need not be so strong. Even though we are rightly cautioned that we have only the most modest of tools and must not extend ourselves too far and though I have myself long advocated such caution, I now believe it is no longer possible to delay using such knowledge as we have in an attempt—feeble and fluttering though it prove itself—to understand and contribute to the control of the social forces which threaten to engulf and enslave us. I was impressed by the frequency with which Bertrand Russell in a recent essay [18] mentioned psychology as a tool for elucidating this or that social force (the control of aggression, for instance) or expressed the hope that it could help in solving a number of problems.

The psychiatrist [19] has prized his knowledge of the individual; he has almost turned his back on the knowledge of social reality, much of which, to be sure, stems from disciplines other than our own. But by now the concept of a dichotomy between the individual and society has worn so thin as to no longer offer even a suitable rationalization for our failure to study social phenomena. A group is something more than the sum of its constituent individuals and increasingly we sense the need of a developing science of group behavior. A society is a continuum and all behavior is bio-psycho-social.

A primary need for us psychiatrists is a proper estimate of social dangers. These dangers may be direct threats to life or limb or they may represent frustration of basic personality needs. These needs may relate to security strivings, pleasure drives or sexual expression, or they may represent aspects of the strivings for self-fulfillment in society. If such danger and frustration are excessive, the adaptive energies of the person may be absorbed in the negative task of counteracting such threats. In such instances, the pathological defense reactions of the personality may be so strongly mobilized as to leave the positive aspects of emotional living and self fulfillment relatively impoverished.[20]

It is necessary that the psychiatrist not only understand the individual and his development but have a concept of social organization as well. In other words, we need a concept—an "ideal" if you will—for normalcy in social structure as well as in the individual. As I have said, whether we admit it or not, in our everyday psychotherapeutic work with patients, we are continually applying an ideal of "normal" both for the individual and for the social environment. In making choices among available alternatives we must be guided by an awareness of the goal we want to reach. In the absence of goals (values), action becomes reduced to emphasizing exclusively the immediate present which is clearly no basis for a sound society.

The concept of "normal" is still far from clear as applied to the individual; it is much less understood as it refers to social structure. Here psychiatry must await in good part the help of other social scientists and participate in collaborative efforts designed to shed new light in this obscure field.

All this grows in importance when we attempt to translate knowledge of human behavior into social action. The application of such knowledge to society is qualified by our own value judgments. These serve as a motivational base for the execution of social responsibility and are the immediate incentive for social action.

An individual learns much about the conflict in his values through his action in and reaction to a group program. I have seen this clearly in my own activities and those of other psychiatrists in connection with what are usually called "action programs." As soon as we are confronted with the need to leave the secluded protection of the study and treatment room and join with people interested in getting things done, or at least started, activities which demand re-examination and probably some shifts in our values, an immense amount of anxiety and insecurity is engendered. May I give you an example of what I mean. The Committee on Social Issues of the Group for the Advancement of Psychiatry proposed a resolution endorsing the Report of the President's Commission on Civil Rights. We had thought this innocent enough and a highly appropriate step for a group of forward-looking psychiatrists. We were literally dismayed at the intense feeling it generated in the group and the hostility and defensiveness which developed as a reaction to the anxiety. The issues involved (in general, prejudice and discrimination against minority groups and the various manifestations of such discrimination) are clearly based in good part on value judgments; the first impact of the resolution was a reaction against this assault on ancient and treasured value systems. It is only fair to add that the opportunity for contemplation and discussion led to the resolution of such conflicts and that the proposed statement was later unanimously passed by the group. This clash in values is part of the process of healthy adaptation. The capacity to effect shifts in values is immeasurably strengthened through group participation and cohesion.

Values represent our orientation to society and our attitude toward human welfare. *In the last analysis, adjustment is a name for the process of living up to a set of values.*

Russell comments that the United States is a country, in the words of the Great Emancipator, "dedicated to a proposition." In the social crises that menace us, we must make a most earnest effort to gain greater knowledge and to apply whatever knowledge we have, partial and sketchy though it is, to counteract social danger and promote healthier living both for individuals and for groups. This may require us to relinquish roles in which we feel secure for ventures far afield; to deny this necessity would be, in truth, to deny those values we most dearly cherish.

Following the completion of this essay, I happened on a quotation which I feel is so apt that I should like to add it: "On a group of theories, one can found a school; on a group of values, one can found a culture, a civilization, a new way of living together among men." [21]

6. RELIGION AND PSYCHIATRY

PERHAPS the very first question that is posed by an effort to survey the relationship between religion and psychiatry grows out of what seems the continuing assumption of an almost inevitable opposition between the two. Despite all the efforts, publicized and otherwise, to create a harmonious relation between religion and psychiatry, there persists a deep and widespread hostility, shared by many if not most of the practitioners of both.[1]

When we consider that psychiatry is a branch of medicine, it is strange to find such persistent expressions of disagreement. Originally medicine and religion had been so closely related as to be inseparable. The magic power to promote human welfare, to avert wrath, to purify streams, to prevent epidemics, to increase fertility and potency—these were shared in earlier days by god and sorcerer, priest and physician. It has often been pointed out that such healers as the Shaman of antiquity was priest, prophet, and medical man and that in fact many of the devices he and other early healers used were closely allied to autosuggestive procedures, and hence a sort of psychotherapy.

Of all the branches of medicine, psychiatry with its philosophical preoccupations with the nature of evil and its concern with supernatural influences on the behavior of man seemed closest to religion. Earlier, it shared with religion the concern for the cure of men's souls; as late as the middle of the nineteenth century a German psychiatrist, Heinroth, expressing his opposition to the increasing spirit of narrow somatology, declaimed: "Soul, the great, most meaningful word! The only treasure of man, the very being of self. How they drag you down by making you the slave of the body." Indeed, he and his contemporaries were accused of speaking "like theologians."

With the rise of materialism and the development of the natural sciences, a head-on clash between religion and science was inevitable. These were the days of self-consciously and violently espoused atheism, the time when it was energetically prophesied that science with its myriad of new discoveries had ended the need for religion and would surely effect the end of the church. Bitter and eloquent denunciations of religion were declaimed and the library of the new "religion" of science grew apace. Psychiatry, too, moved on from its earlier preoccupations with sin and evil and renounced its beliefs in demons, unplacated gods, and other magical causes for emotional and mental illness. As it moved along with general medical science in the direction of detailed observation and the development of new instruments of scientific precision for the study of tissue and body processes, psychiatry became increasingly absorbed in "objective" science, and retreated from a position closely akin to religion to a sort of total immersion in the quest for organic elements in disease and a tremendous concern with the description and classification of diseases.

A corrective was not long in coming. Under the impact of the development of psychoanalysis, psychiatry turned sharply—perhaps too sharply—from its concern with disturbed tissues to the explanation of human emotional illness in purely psychological terms. Now the emphasis was on early life experience and parent-child relations and the word "love" was again abroad in mental science.

While much of the responsibility for the clash between religion and psychiatry may be attributed to the general rise of scientific materialism, there is no question in my mind that by far the greatest impetus to this conflict stems from Freud's attitude toward religion and his attacks on it, especially his classical diatribe, "The Future of an Illusion." To appreciate the impact of this and other works on religion which Freud published would require a much fuller discussion than is possible or appropriate in this place. However, some discussion of his criticism is imperative.

But perhaps before I undertake this, I should pause for some general reflections and definitions. Religion is fabulously difficult to define and yet without some such attempt, it is almost impossible to discuss these matters at all. The definitions range from the so-called "minimum" definition used by anthropologists, "The belief in spiritual beings," through Frazier's widely quoted, "A propitiation or conciliation of powers superior to man which are believed to direct and control the course of nature and of human life." There is the widely recalled definition of Donald Hankey, devised in the trenches of World War I: "Religion is betting your life there is a God" (which recalls its World War II counterpart: "There are no atheists in foxholes").

More important, perhaps, than an effort at precise definition, is the recognition of the important role which religion plays in the life of man. Too often, the irreligious person responds to any discussion of religion by evoking a tried and trusted stereotype: some cherished prejudice, a partial or cloudy memory of some church ritual or a childhood deprivation or punishment inflicted by a parent in the name of religion. This preoccupation with the mechanical minu-tiae of religious form serves to deny its role in the general life experience of people, its place as an essential element in the universal need to find answers to the inevitable questions of whither, whence, and why which disturb, confuse, and challenge all of us. As Herskovits comments, "However he defines the universe, man everywhere uses religion *to find and maintain himself in the scheme of things* [My italics]. Religion, like all other aspects of life, is a functioning ele-ment of culture."

There is a rather general tendency to equate religion with an institution, a particular church or sect and, indeed, to carry this even further, to a particular place of worship. On the other hand, there is also the tendency to discard en-tirely the institutional and formal aspects of religion in an attempt to distill the essence of it into a body of ethical and moral principles or rules of conduct. To be sure, an ethic is basic to a religion and in our culture all religions are vitally concerned with the promulgation of "rules" for living. However, there is a vital and necessary distinction to be made between a religion and its moral and ethical compo-nents. Religion goes beyond moral and ethical concepts; it is a body of shared beliefs, ceremonials, and practices which symbolize for the religious the heart of their common faith. Religion requires active participation, not the pas-sivity which is peculiarly a manifestation of contemporary life: "in professing our faith, we lend our presence and our ears but not a hand. The immediate relevance of belief to action, so essential a characteristic of religion in most cul-tures, seems, somehow to be absent." (Herskovits.)

Universal in any definition of religion is the concept of *faith*, but this hardly advances our quest for a definition since the word itself is used in so many ways. It was Oliver Wendell Holmes who said that "the great act of faith is

when man decides that he is not God." The classic definition of faith remains that of the writer of the epistle to the
Hebrews, who declared that "faith is . . . the evidence of
things not seen." It is obvious that faith is basic in many
more things than in religion, although certainly and emphatically it is at the root of religious belief. To take but one
example: think of friendship and human love without faith;
it is truly inconceivable, and, as in religion, it is so generally
accepted as to rarely require any explicit acknowledgment.

I shall use religion to mean those beliefs of man concerning his relation to the unknown (nature and God) which
have an institutionalized form: a tradition, a church, a system of law, a priesthood, ceremonials, and sacraments. For
Freud, religion "consists of certain dogmas, assertions about
facts and conditions of external (or internal) reality, which
tell one something that one has not oneself discovered and
which claim that one should give them credence."

Freud considered religion a manifestation of man's feelings of helplessness and the continuation of a type of solution which the infant uses to try to ward off his understandable feelings of defenselessness, i.e., the dependence on a
strong adult (father) figure and a clinging to that figure for
support. And so, he says, "a rich store of ideas is formed,
born of the need to make tolerable the helplessness of man
and built out of the material offered by memories of the
helplessness of his own childhood and the childhood of the
human race. It is easy to see that these ideas protect man in
two directions: against the dangers of nature and fate and
against the evils of human society itself." And, he continues,
"now that God is a single person, man's relation to Him
could recover the intimacy and intensity of the child's relation to the father. If one had done so much for the father,
then surely one would be rewarded—at least the beloved
child, the chosen people would be." (As an example of the

need to be the only beloved child, Freud comments: "Pious America has laid claim to be God's own country.")

Of course, Freud knew that men, always and everywhere, have been and still are preoccupied with questions to which science and naturalism have as yet offered no satisfactory answers: why we are, whence we come, what is the meaning of life, and our destiny after death. Even he had acknowledged "the painful riddle of death, for which no remedy at all has yet been found *nor probably ever will be.*" (My italics).

In essence, what Freud objected to in religion was its fostering of man's dependent relation to a superior, more powerful figure, God, the omnipotent father; an attitude which he feared might prevent man from maturing into a healthy independence. For Freud, religious ideas were illusions and "culture incurs a greater danger by maintaining its present attitude toward religion than by relinquishing it." Most curious and difficult to understand is Freud's blaming religion for failing to make mankind happy; "we see an appallingly large number of men discontented with civilization and unhappy with it." This from Freud, who elsewhere had warned of the utter inevitability of what he termed "the everyday unhappiness" of man.

I must refrain from any attempt to analyze in any detail this crucial contribution of Freud. Herskovits' estimate of it seems reasonable enough: "The Freudian explanation of religion, in terms of the unconscious desire for the security of childhood, where a parent, as surrogate for society, solved problems and made decisions as well as directed conduct, is too simple to be fully acceptable; but it does give us an important insight into probable motivations that lead to religious expression."

Which brings me suitably to what I consider a major defect in Freud's contention about religion: his failure to make explicit and examine in this connection the difference between motivation and behavior. Zilboorg has pointed out that "some ingenious critic of empirical and experimental science might . . . turn the tables and say, not entirely without right and plausibility, that science ought to be rejected because it is an outlet for man's inordinate infantile, peeping, sexual curiosity, because it is merely a formalized expression of his faith in himself and in his ultimate mastery over nature and man." In this connection I am reminded of an atomic scientist I had in treatment for whom the elaborate and extremely complicated machinery with which he dealt was, in his unconscious, the ultimate fulfillment of his need for power, indeed for omnipotence. Actually, he was a weak, timid man, socially seclusive, terrified by women, and lost in constant reverie of his as yet undemonstrated sexual prowess. His science, however, was superb; his contribution to basic research recognized and rewarded. Now, one would hardly despise scientific labors because of their unconscious roots in infantile needs; why then should one not at least be willing to examine religion in terms, so to speak, of its deeds?

I do not wish to strain this analogy nor in any way to deprecate the importance of the historic fact that there are great evils inherent in the authoritarian church and that the pages of history are bloody with the ravages of wars conducted in the name of religion. To do this would be ignorant and false; in addition, it would lead me to an attempted defense of the worst of religious practices—a task for which I would have no stomach. Besides, I believe it to be irrelevant to this discussion.

For me the nature (the fact) of religion is one of values. Surely no one is more aware than psychoanalysts that values have their roots in childhood experiences. The inevitable feeling of helplessness which all children experience requires an opportunity for identification, for security-yielding love relations, and for opportunities for the healthy life experiences of childhood which are the road to emotional well-being. This is a psychoanalytic axiom; why then is it necessary that healthy religious experience and the formation of high religious values be excluded from the general rules and customs of living which ideally result in other sound attitudes and values? To be sure, we must carefully scrutinize such processes and not exempt certain religious attitudes and practices from the necessity for change. But neither can we exclude all religious acts as though they inevitably resulted in warped attitudes and crippling experiences, as though religion were the absolute and certain concomitant of neurotic helplessness and sick dependence. To be sure, many psychiatrists and psychoanalysts believe this; it is the more surprising therefore, how little discussion there has been on the subject by these practitioners, how automatic this conclusion has become and how sedulously—one might say "religiously"—maintained. There are some notable exceptions: in the work of Fromm, for whom religion is essentially the equivalent of a benign and progressive ethical system; of Karl Menninger, for whom it is a matter essentially of faith; and of Gregory Zilboorg, who to my knowledge has published the only critical estimate of the traditional Freudian approach. For Zilboorg religion is an integral part of our cultural existence and growth and he sees both religion and psychoanalysis seeking "to solve the difficult problems which impose themselves upon man in his constant state of anxiety and sense of guilt." He comments: "Both seek the path that would lead to serenity and attenuation of the sense of guilt. Each uses a terminology of its own but both seem to have solved the problem on the basis of the same principle. Both give the principle the same name —love."

Much of this attempt to reconcile religion and psychiatry suggests a "therapeutic" role for the former as an important if not indeed its main function. To be sure the creative power, the healing strength, the comforting balm of religion are well known and for the believer a great and abiding strength. And many a purported disbeliever has eagerly turned to religion when faced with the overwhelming threat of a crisis in his life or the impact of personal tragedy and grief.

But it is essential that we look beyond this role if we are to understand the true meaning and importance of religion. For long centuries the Jewish and Christian traditions have been the main source of man's ordering of his values and the need for high, shared and firmly established values has perhaps never been greater than now. This need must have much to do with the increase in formal religious practice as well as the acknowledged return of intellectuals to religion. A recent symposium in the *Partisan Review* stems from the position that "one of the most significant tendencies of our time, especially in this decade, has been the new turning toward religion among intellectuals and the growing disfavor with which secular attitudes and perspectives are now regarded in not a few circles that lay claim to the leadership of culture." A surprising array of intellectuals who contributed to that symposium acknowledged this fact, whatever else their disagreements were.

One or two instances of issues which are of common concern to both psychiatrists and religious thinkers must suffice. Man is always confronted with basic conflicts between current pleasures and successful planning for the future which often require the postponement of satisfactions. In adolescence, for instance, such problems are of the greatest concern. It is well known that the individual is enabled to achieve the necessary postponement of satisfaction because he has what is called technically a strong ego; the roots of this are in a healthy childhood and an opportunity for the child to learn the need for sharing and for postponement of the immediate demands for satisfaction. Religion has always stressed the importance of living not for the moment but for the future; modern dynamic psychiatry changes the language but mirrors the exact sentiment.

Or take the problems of loyalty, the devotion to friend, school, cause, or country. Psychoanalysis has in this instance confirmed what was known from antiquity. Religious thinkers have long emphasized the necessity to understand one's obligations and responsibilities to others beyond the immediate hope of gain and reward for oneself. To survive, man must be egotistical; to mature, he must be something more than egotistical. Much of this thinking is now reflected in everyday "child guidance" principles without ever a thought to the extent to which religious values are involved in such principles and, indeed, are available to strengthen their inculcation. Similarly, with group activity. The importance of such activities for both the maturing child and the adult is constantly and properly emphasized in psychological writing. Religious devotion was always centered on group activity even though the right of the individual was always equally respected. The close relationship of the synagogue, for instance, with communal living, with the education of the young and with the regulation of civil affairs, illustrates a type of group adherence and solidarity which can be applauded even when viewed in the most sophisticated psychological terms.

For those who would demolish religion, science is usually advanced as its rational and sound substitute. This was also true for Freud: "The more the fruits of knowledge become accessible to men, the more widespread is the decline of religious belief." In an age where science has been responsible for loosening the bonds of atomic energy and the scientifically devised instruments of war which grow ever more terrifying, the defense of science as a substitute for religious values would be a perilous undertaking. I do not mean to oversimplify this problem and appear to assume what would be a naïve and unrealistic attitude toward the necessity for the utilization of science for defense, although one distinguished American scientist has, indeed, refused to make available any of his research which he thought could be put to military purposes. Even Freud was not too certain of the efficacy of his "cure" for religion and could admit that perhaps in science he too was "chasing after an illusion. Perhaps the effect of religious thought prohibition is not as bad as I assume; perhaps it will turn out that human nature remains the same even if education is not abused by being subjected to religion."

But why "abused"? Modern education for healthy emotional development places great stress on such things as early identification patterns, the acquisition of sound values, the capacity to withstand the everyday frustrations and disappointments of life, the necessity for shared living, the crucial role of the ability to love and be loved. Each of these and many other such concepts are now better understood because of the development of modern psychological science (and we must never forget that it is to Freud that by far the greatest credit for this must surely go!). But these goals have always been part of the ancient teachings of religion, especially of the Jewish and Christian teachings of the Western world, and we know that religion can provide vitally rich and lasting tools to help achieve the goals of modern education.

Cardinal Newman said, "In religious inquiry each of us can speak only for himself" and in that spirit I venture to speak of some of my own religious experiences. Thus I re-

member with deep affection and gratitude the beauty of
the Sabbath in my home; my mother's unlettered but
devout observances and the way the children were permitted to share and learn; the rich ceremonials and the
joyous occasions of the festival day observances; the aura
of peace and security which we children all felt as a holiday
shut out of our home the insecurities and travail of "everyday unhappiness." I believe such practices are in keeping
with the best psychiatric formulations, though I would
hardly wish to tarnish my memory of them by any such
"scientific" rationale.

How about the other side of the coin? For instance, the
fanatic love- and pleasure-depriving injunctions of certain
religions, or the obsessional characteristics of certain observances? In the first place, it must be recognized that there
is nothing in religion per se which indicts corporal love-
making or the pursuit of happiness. In general it may be said
that for most religions the emphasis is only on moderation,
on the preservation of the family unit, on the avoidance of
the perverse and extreme, all of which psychiatry would
heartily echo. For a Jew, for instance, virtue is a pleasure.
There is no place for wanton sensuality, but neither is the
human body considered corrupt or degraded. In the old
ghettos on a Friday night the pious Jew would perfume
himself and comb his hair before he went to prayer, would
fervently chant the Song of Songs at the table, and, after
the Sabbath supper, the best meal of the week, he generally
went to bed with his wife. Nothing harsh or repressive or
denying in this, or, for that matter, nothing not consonant
with modern psychological thinking!

Of the traditional notion that religious people can't have
fun, that religion is principally a system of taboos designed
to make men and women unhappy, Headley says "it is as
meaningless as the still enduring American superstition that

no Englishman has a sense of humour . . . Where there is
no reason against pleasure, then pleasure is authentically a
fulfillment of the wholeness of the Christian life." And of
the Sabbath, scripture says, "This is the day which the Lord
hath made; we will rejoice and be glad in it."

What of the accusation that religious practices are "obsessional"? For some people they truly are, just as for some
others "religion" takes on the coloration of psychotic delusions. One should neither condemn religion because of the
person who believes his religious instruction comes directly
to him through the spoken word of the Lord [2] nor find
fault with it because some religious people, terrified and
helpless, attempt to find sanctuary in endless repetitive, compulsive patterns of religious ceremonial. These are matters of
individual adjustment or maladjustment and I doubt that
one is any more entitled to draw conclusions from such
illustrations than one would be to criticize science because,
as is well known, many scientists are extremely compulsive,
as, for that matter, are butchers, bakers, and candlestick
makers.

Paul Tillich in an eloquent passage has said that there are
only two approaches to the predicament of the modern
world: the negative-religious and the positive-religious. The
former he calls the way of despair and heroism ("its heroism
is the acceptance of its despair"). The positive-religious
way transcends the human predicament radically by trans-
forming it into a question to which religion gives the answer. He goes on to say: "Religion is *not* a collection of
theoretical statements of a questionable or superstitious
character. Such a religion could not be accepted by an intellectual who is not willing to sacrifice his intellectual
honesty. Some of them make this sacrifice and surrender
their intellectual autonomy to Ecclesiastical or Biblical authorities. But their turn to religion is still an expression of

their despair, not a victory over it. Others are waiting for a religious answer which does not destroy reason but points to the mystery in the ground of the natural, which denies that God is a being and speaks of Him as the ground and depth of being and meaning, which knows about the significance of symbols in myth and cult, but resists the distortion of symbols into statements of knowledge which necessarily conflict with scientific knowledge. A theology which takes this position, which preserves the intellectual honesty of the intellectual and expresses, at the same time, the answers to the questions implied in man's existence and existence generally—such a theology is acceptable to the intelligentsia (and to many non-intellectuals as well). It prevents the turn of the intellectuals toward religion from becoming a matter of romantic concessions or of self-surrender to authority."

With such a theology, psychiatry can have no basic conflict; in the quest for values that can give support and strength and a sense of the beauty and meaning of life, each can contribute richly from its store of learning and belief.

II. Psychiatry and Social Issues

7. CULTURAL FACTORS IN SOCIAL WORK

SOCIAL WORK'S interest in culture is relatively recent; and in this social work merely reflects a rapidly growing trend.[1] This has been accelerated by the fact that anthropology has turned increasingly to a concern with culture as an entity and recently has given more and more attention to the study of contemporary people.

It will not be my purpose to enter into any detailed discussion of the theory and application of "culturology." This is a highly technical branch of knowledge, confessedly beyond my scope, and I have leaned almost entirely for the preparation of this material on the generally known published works of such distinguished writers in the field as Benedict, Mead, and especially Herskovits, whose textbook *Man and His Works* is particularly suited to students in other fields who desire to inform themselves of the general field of anthropology and its most recent approaches to the study of culture. It is a book I earnestly recommend.

For present purposes I would simply like to set forth in a preliminary way a number of propositions concerning culture. But first we need a usable definition, and there are many to choose from. One of the best definitions is E. B. Taylor's,[2] who described culture as "the complex whole that includes knowledge, belief, art, morals, law, custom and any other capabilities and habits acquired by man as a member of society." Herskovits' [3] definition is also appropriate:

Culture is the man-made part of the environment. Implicit in this is the recognition that man's life is lived in a dual setting, the natural habitat and his social "environment." The definition also implies that culture is more than a biological phenomenon. It includes all the elements in man's mature endowment that he has acquired from his group by conscious learning or, on a somewhat different level, by a conditioning process—techniques of various kinds, social and other institutions, beliefs, and patterned needs of conduct.

The first proposition we would emphasize is: culture is the *learned* portion of human behavior. The key word here is "learned" for, as Herskovits states, "it is recognized by all students that whatever forms susceptible of objective description may compose a culture, they must be learned by succeeding generations of a population if they are not to be lost." [4] We can study "culture" as a phenomenon but, to the people who live in it, culture is the composite of the things that they have, do, think, and believe. Of the first importance is the fact that culture is learned both at the conscious level, through education of all sorts, and also at an unconscious level, whereby the basic patterns of the group are impressed on the developing infant. The latter is of fundamental consequence.

The process of learning one's culture is called "enculturation." It is through this process that a culture maintains a recognizable form generation after generation. Every individual is born into a group whose customs and beliefs are established *before* he comes on the scene. Actually, we learn the lessons of our culture so well that much of our later behavior is automatic response to certain stimuli. Of course, this transmission belt is not meant to imply a rigidity and steadfastness in the process that does not allow for change. Every society accepts variations in modes of behavior. In every culture there is room for change; were that not so, man would be but a creature of his culture without choice or the possibility of altering life situations "imposed" by his culture.

One of the most striking and familiar evidences of such change, and one within the knowledge of us all, is the amazing shift in cultural patterns of behavior which was achieved by many (but not by all!) of the European escapees to this country. I have commented elsewhere [5] on this and other similar shifts in connection with some reflections on the subject of values, but the illustration is equally pertinent in this consideration of culture.

Values are themselves derived from the culture and might well be included in the "complex whole" which Taylor used to define culture. As we shall see, many of the problems that are said to derive from conflicts between cultural patterns can perhaps best be described and understood in terms of values.

A necessary distinction, perhaps especially so for social workers, is the one between culture and society, since social work is still so largely concerned with the "social" aspects of life. Again to follow Herskovits: "A culture is the way of life of a people, while a society is the organized aggregates of individuals who follow a given way of life." In simpler terms: "A society is composed of people; the way they behave is their culture."

It may appear that this distinction is tenuous and too highly theoretical to have much usefulness for the present discussion, and from a practical, work-a-day point of view this is possibly true. However, these are valid distinctions and should help us achieve a more precise use of the concept of culture.

Man [6] is the only creature that has achieved culture—that is, whose ways of meeting demands are cumulative and much more varied than those of any other species in the biological series.[7]

Actually, whatever the distinctions, there is a close parallelism between social and cultural life and perhaps it suffices for our purposes to remember that the latter term is the broader, including as it does certain aspects of behavior such as religion, the arts, language, and the unspoken sanctions that underlie all conduct, which are not included in the term *social*.[8]

It follows then that man is the only culture-building animal, though not the only *social* animal. This societal quality among the lower animals is now well known and has been described for a whole range of animals from ants to the baboons.[9] But man is the only *speaking* animal and therein rests his power of continuously changing his way of life through the invention and accumulation of new habits, passed on from generation to generation by the *verbal* symbols of language.[10] An adequate discussion of this relation of symbols (language) to culture would take us far afield.

A second and fundamental proposition concerning culture is the fact that understanding of a culture requires an understanding of the individual. No fundamental comprehension of culture can be achieved that leaves the individual out of account. Thus psychology, which is concerned essentially with the study of the individual, joins anthropology to enlighten us about culture. All psychology, and especially psychoanalysis, is concerned with the genetic process, the way in which the individual develops from his beginnings, and it thus emphasizes his earliest life experiences. Anthropology demonstrates how these experiences are culturally determined. In the study of Travelers Aid clients which follows, we shall try to emphasize the contributions from both fields, which together will help us to comprehend the whole situation more adequately.

One of the common confusions in the understanding of the cultural process is around the meaning of race. This naturally becomes a matter of primary significance for us in the social sciences since the distortion of the significance of race has been and still is to put to the service of bias and prejudice in an all too familiar pattern. As Herskovits emphasizes: "Race has never been satisfactorily proved to influence culture." [11] It has been demonstrated again and again that there is no scientific validity in any of the racist philosophies and that "any child of ordinary capacity whatever his racial affiliation can be enculturated to any way of life."

Naturally, physical type and culture are related, and cultural factors influence physical type. There is the social selection of mates, diet, occupations, and child-rearing practices, all of which influence individual characteristics and are rooted in the culture.

A most important aspect of culture is that it is *dynamic*, that *change* is a constant in human culture. However, alongside of this it should be emphasized that cultures are basically very stable, i.e., that these changes seldom affect more than a relatively small part of the total body of custom by which people live. This despite the fact that the changes may seem tremendous to the members of a particular society in which they are taking place. Such changes can come from within a society, through discovery or invention, or from without through a selective form of borrowing.

Culture is a variable, which is an expression of its dynamic quality. There are two types of variation—first in human culture as a whole, the ways different people have decided to achieve the same ends, and second the variation that is expressed in the differences in behavior of individual members of the same society. In this connection, it should be noted that in small social units, as in the family, there is less tendency for variation in its members.

Much of what has been learned about culture has been derived from the study of primitive and remote peoples. It is really only in the last ten years or so, under the inspired leadership of Benedict, Mead, and their co-workers, that anthropology has turned its attention to the study of contemporary peoples and culture, and of the cultural character structure. The methodology of these studies is extremely interesting; we can only mention here its inter-disciplinary nature, drawing as it does on cultural anthropology, clinical psychology, child development, psycho-analysis, history, ecology, etc. These studies have provided us with a rich and varied literature, some of which will be used in our discussion of particular cases. A study of a reasonable sampling of this material is highly recommended.[12]

One of the most relevant and important abstractions which we can draw from this approach is that of culture and character structure. In this context, culture is used to mean "the total shared learned behavior of a functioning autonomous society over a time span that includes many generations." The concept of cultural character structure denotes the "regularities in the intrapsychic organization of the individual members of a given society that are to be attributed to these individuals having been reared within that culture."[13] Mead goes on to say:

In the study of culture, the behaviour of individuals is examined in order to make statements about the shared culture that are of such a nature that they can be discussed without invoking any specific theory of learning or of psychodynamics.

It will be important for us to remember that "culture is the instrument whereby the individual adjusts to his total setting and gains the means for creative expression." [14]

It might be well to begin with a consideration of the six clients of Travelers Aid who are American Indians since they illustrate the whole range of the effect of culture on the client, the worker, and the casework process.

The first case concerns a Navajo Indian couple. The man's family was wealthy as reckoned in Navajoland but his wife came from a poverty-stricken home. Both are Baptists and devoted to some of the missionaries who work with the Indians. Lena, the wife, has been known to the agency since 1944, but the reasons for this initial contact are not stated. She is described as "of fine character, a reliable worker, and personally very neat." Lena had lived with white people during her youth; she loved her life with them but yearned for the reservation whenever she was away from it.

This couple sought Travelers Aid help for a host of problems, in what appears to have been a quest for a generally supporting, friendly relationship. The record states: "Any emergency is likely to bring Ray and Lena to the agency."

Of particular significance are the comments of the caseworkers, themselves born and reared in the Southwest of parents who were greatly interested in Indian welfare. The workers appear to have been accepted "more as the clients' own people." We shall return to discuss the advantages and disadvantages of this type of matching of worker and client in connection with another case. With the Indians some of the advantages are manifest. For instance, it is emphasized that "the long silences of Ray and

Lena do not mean rejection of advice offered but more likely a careful pondering of it. It can also be the comfortable silence of a deeply felt friendship for the worker. Indians also size up strangers during a prolonged silence since they do not find silences awkward or embarrassing as do most white people."

I was especially interested in the workers' comment that the "interviews must be slow-paced and can be maddening when other cases need attention." Every so often, I visit a hospital where the patient population is largely drawn from rural, mountaineer people. In the first few interviews on each visit I am extremely uncomfortable; I find it almost impossible to wait for answers to my questions and must make a conscious effort to adapt my pace to the leisurely tempo of my patients. As with the Indian clients, this slow pace in speaking does not reflect pathology but cultural patterns of speech and contemplation.

The importance to the patient or client of the therapist's or caseworker's ability to recognize such differences and make the necessary adjustment to the situation will be apparent. Interruptions are almost inevitably interpreted as hostility or indifference.[15]

Another factor of interest concerns budgeting, which these Indian clients find difficult if not impossible to do. They are apparently accustomed to barter rather than cash purchases, as so many of their transactions have been with the traders. Thus, Ray could not comprehend the to him complicated finances of the purchase of a car "on time" and quickly lost it because of inability to maintain his payments. This is, of course, a common enough experience but in reading the record it seemed quite clear that the dilemma was the result not of improvidence or stupidity but of a failure to comprehend the meaning of a social pattern that was strange and unfamiliar. He could not accept the fact that the car would be repossessed; after all, he protested, he had "already paid a lot on the car." The record comments: "Again the attitude was due to dealings with the traders, who endeavor to accommodate Indians."

As Indians have always had free medical and hospital care on the reservation, the first doctor bill and the cost of medicine were a shock to Lena and Ray. Another factor that made a hospital experience troublesome for Lena was what she considered unseemly haste in reaching the decision to hospitalize her. As in other situations in their lives, they, as Indians, required a lot of time to contemplate the problem and reach a suitable conclusion. Lena's relationship with a public agency worker who had no knowledge of Indians intensified her difficulties, especially as this worker never could wait long enough for a thoughtful response and seemed intolerant of Lena's long periods of silence. Finally Lena "walked out" of the hospital, presumably to go visit her children. It turned out that she had actually run away so that she could consult a tribal medicine man. "All her experience in early youth in our hospitals and with our doctors could not break the old tribal faith in medicine men." She had consulted one of the type known as "a shaker." The record states, rather plaintively, I thought: "He shook a handful of sacred meal in the air and came up with the comforting diagnosis: 'You don't have tuberculosis.'" It is understandable that Lena resents the compulsory visits to clinics or from the public health nurse, which are, to say the least, remarkably different from her "treatments" by the medicine man.

A further problem was precipitated when it was necessary for them to place their children in school. Lena and Ray had gone only to Indian schools and were frankly distrustful of the unknown. It required excellent and understanding casework to overcome this culturally rooted apprehension, especially since it had been fortified by experience with hostile, prejudiced white children in another community. The school problem was indeed complicated for both the children and parents by incidents of physical harm inflicted by some of the Negro children. These and other manifestations of prejudice reappear often throughout the record. We shall return to this point in connection with another case but we might note here one of the cruelest and most basic aspects of prejudice: the need of each group, no matter how greatly it has itself suffered the results of prejudice, to find victims in the members of another group on which it can, in turn, vent its hostility.

Throughout the record, however, we find mention of problems which seem quite unrelated to the fact that Lena and Ray are Indians. Ray's very occasional "drunk," the worries about money, concern for the children's health, all seem the ordinary problems of parents with no economic security and no deep roots in any community. It is always difficult, though, to draw any clear line of demarcation between what is "cultural" and what is not and, in the end, it seems not too useful to try to draw such subtle distinctions. We need to remember that the individual reflects his cultural background to some measure in every aspect of his personality and adjustment and that these distinctions are often only matters of emphasis.

A second case involving Indians is that of Mrs. Whiteheel. A 45-year-old "old fashioned "squaw-type of Indian woman—hair hanging in braids, slovenly in dress though warmly clothed in a good coat"—had left the reservation despite the fact that she was in the last weeks of pregnancy, leaving three children and a mother on relief. She and her husband had set out to find more remunerative employment but had become intoxicated and wound up in a neighboring jail. She was impatient with any offer or effort to help and wanted only to get her husband out of jail so that they might start to hitchhike again. She knew that she might deliver at any moment, had made no preparations whatsoever for the baby, and showed absolutely no concern about this. She said "he" (her husband) would take care of everything; "when 'he' gets out (of jail) he'll get whatever I need." She refused the offer of a cab back to the shelter from the agency office, "snorted," and said: "Don't waste any money on a cab for me—I can walk back" (at least 20 blocks).

Of considerable relevancy and interest is this paragraph in the record:

Suddenly Mrs. Whiteheel dived into her large pocket in the full skirt she was wearing and produced a paper sack containing samples of exquisite bead weaving, bracelets lined with chamois-skin, bootees, etc. Her facial expression changed for the first time and she actually smiled as she showed the worker her handiwork.

The worker adds laconically: "at the end of the interview Mrs. W. said she felt fine." Mr. W. was soon released from jail and they disappeared.

I would like to quote the worker's evaluation in full:

The cultural pattern of this couple's background is reflected in the carefree manner in which they "struck out" from the reservation; the dependence of Mrs. Whiteheel on "him" and her complete trust in "his" ability to see them through; her stolid facing of unpleasant facts; her indifference to physical discomfort and pain; her scorn of medical care in a minor incident such as childbirth; her pleasure in her own talent for handiwork which she proudly said she learned at "the school"; her acceptance, as a matter of course, of the fact that her husband "threw a big one" when they got drunk together; her casual attitude about clothing for the baby. The one false note was her willingness to leave her three children and her philosophical remark that "she didn't have them with her anyway."

A first reading of this case record left me with the feeling that we were dealing with a psychopathic personality, possibly in a mentally retarded woman. To take off from "home" in the last weeks of pregnancy, deserting three children, without any plans except a vague hope for her husband's employment in a distant, unknown city, with no arrangement or supplies for her expected child; to get drunk and end up in jail; to refuse help of any kind—this is certainly a familiar enough pattern of behavior, and ordinarily we would consider it "sick," whatever specific diagnosis we attached to it.

But is this clinical insight enough? Frankly my knowledge of the American Indian is too limited to have anything approaching an authoritative view, but a few things seem certain. We have apparently infantilized these people, making them totally dependent and hence completely improvident. Then, how much of her "revolt" might well be part of a general if inappropriate and disproportionate reaction to hostility, prejudice, and deprivation? Can we speak of a reservation as "home," especially when at home all her children are away, two at school (is this by choice or necessity?) and the youngest, a 17-month-old baby, still in a hospital?

Rather, I think, we have here a case that illustrates very well the constant interplay between cultural and personal factors, in which certain attitudes are plainly rooted in cultural determinants, but where the "sickness," the personality distortion, represents the individual's failure at adaptation. In this sense, the manifestations are beyond explanation entirely in cultural terms but the bases for such deviation stem from both the early personal and environmental influences and get played out in ways that are at least influenced by the client's cultural background.

In still another case involving an Indian, this time a 15-year-old boy who left his home city to look for his father, there are similar admixtures of factors which might explain the boy's attitude and behavior. This youngster, a Cherokee, was neglected by his mother, deserted by his father, and wholly ignored by an aunt and uncle who live in the city he had fled. It is understandable that one would attempt to use the fact that he is an Indian to explain his passivity and his ability to keep "mum" even when confronted with emotionally disturbing news. But his behavior seems familiarly adolescent and could be easily duplicated in any neglected, traumatized youngster who took off impulsively looking for his father (protection, strength). We do not have the data on which to speculate as to the meaning to him of his father's desertion and his mother's neglect and promiscuity, but we can be certain that they must have mobilized deep feelings of rejection and hostility to which he reacted in flight.

It seems only natural that I should have found a fair sample of adolescents in the cases at my disposal; adolescents are commonly "running away"—from bad news, bad schools, bad parents—all the badness being, of course, the adolescents' verdict. Among these adolescents are two Indian girls, aged 18 and 19 respectively, who were trying to run away from, among other things, being Indian and all that this meant to them.

It is well known that some of the greatest sources of conflict between parents and adolescents derive from cultural, value conflicts. The constant cry and complaint of the adolescent that the older generation doesn't understand him is mirrored in this instance for Ethel and Peg, our Indian

clients. They believe that being Indian (they are both actually half-breeds) meant inevitable conflicts and rejec-
tions because neither parent really accepted the standards,
customs, gods, etc., of the other's group; that they would
constantly be driven by harsh discipline toward conformity,[16] especially to the old tribal customs; and that they
faced the inevitable dependency which seemingly results
from being Indian, from the things that are done for a person simply because he is Indian.

The problem of dependency and the revolt against it is
characteristic of adolescents of all cultures, reflecting the
more basic need to revolt against being a child and the
struggle to be independent (adult), together with the terror
which the latter prospect holds. Every adolescent is constantly running away psychologically and tries to run away
more literally at least once, even though he actually con-
trives to be discovered even before he has crossed the
threshold. Ethel and Peg needed and received help to recognize that the proverbial grass is not always greener elsewhere and that there is maturity and genuine independence
to be found right in one's own back yard.

A related case is the one of P.C., a 16-year-old boy who
was also a runaway. His parents are Jewish, divorced and
both remarried to Christians. Peter lives with his father and
stepmother; his own mother still lives in Europe. He has
been in the U.S.A. for three years. He could not accept
the discipline of his school and in failing to do so incurred
the hostility of his father, a strict (the record says "German") disciplinarian. (We shall discuss the troublesome
question of stereotypes in connection with a later case.) He
feels rejected by both parents and is in real conflict as to his
religion. He ran away just as he was planning to leave for

Europe to visit his mother, incidentally using money which he had earned and saved. His parents, as one might have expected, were certain that the trouble was simply due to his running around with a "bad crowd" and getting into a mess, thereby confusing cause and result.

The boy is intelligent, "very warm and outgoing." He was contrite on his return, full of promises to turn over a new leaf and cooperate. He was (how characteristic!) most interested in learning if his father had missed him, and when told that he had, said: "This is a happy experience." The record continues: "He explained he felt that his father did not care for him so he felt why should he care."

Thus we have the only too familiar setting and cast of characters: divorced parents, separation from the mother, lack of understanding by the parents and childish provocation by the adolescent, guilt and hostility resulting in abortive, really unwilling flight. In this case the religious conflict probably played a role. Certainly the overpunitive attitude of the father did, whether we think of it as "German" or not. From a considerable clinical experience with children of mixed (Christians and Jews) marriages, I have developed the conviction that in most instances intermarriage adds a severe burden to the universal task faced by all children of developing healthy identification patterns. In many instances, as in this case, the difference in the parents' religions develops in the child feelings of rejection and confusion as to his social role.[17] I have a patient in treatment at this time, the child of Jewish parents, who were divorced when he was five. They both married Christians and all the five children of their subsequent marriages have been raised as Christians. It would be difficult to overemphasize the confusion of roles and identification and the hostility this situation has engendered. Nor are assimilationist attitudes usually more successful, or the device of leaving religion out of the child's life until he is old enough to "make his own choice."

Still another adolescent presents herself for our consideration. An 18-year-old Mexican girl, carrying her clothes in a shopping bag, frightened and lonely, had come to B— to find work. She appeared dull, inexperienced, and very young. She wore a faded but once loud plaid skirt, a sleazy peasant blouse, bobby socks, and extremely large gypsy type earrings. "At this point," the worker knowingly comments, "I realize that Maria who appeared dull, inappropriately dressed, and unattractive to me, *in her own setting* [my italics] would be considered appropriately attired and not too unattractive."

Maria had been born in a Texas border town "where a Mexican was hardly considered a person. She had spent most of her life where there is a definite but inexplicit barrier between the American and Latin American."

Indeed Maria was also running away, trying to be a person in her own right and an adult. What was she attempting to escape? Many things: a notion that she was illegitimate, which proved to be untrue, a father-centered, father-dominated home, a tired, busy, rejecting mother, constant chaperonage,[18] poverty, the appropriation of her pay check, five younger brothers and sisters, insufficient food—a pretty heavy load for a youngster to bear. The worker says: "I began to see Maria as a girl rebelling at the cultural controls of her Latin-American family and anxious to become a modern American." I agree, but this seems too simple; the chaperonage, the father-centeredness of the home, etc., were cultural, but the excesses, the deprivations, and punishments were personal exaggerations, no matter what the cultural sanction may have been. To which was added the inevitable blight of ignorance and poverty, both of which cut cruelly and directly across borders and cultural frontiers. Too often one hears this or that baneful, destructive quality or behavioral pattern characterized as Mexican or Puerto Rican or Jewish when clearly and unmistakably they are the results or at least the concomitants of poverty and ignorance, as are poor housing, bad hygiene, poor health, etc. In this as in others of our cases it is noteworthy that only the negative aspects of the clients' culture are emphasized. The beauty, the traditional strengths, the group affirmations are not mentioned, not because they are absent in the particular culture but because poverty and ignorance and distortions of personal behavior have made them less available and less meaningful. The worker does mention that Maria appreciated art and music, but makes no further comment on these positive factors in the situation.

Maria had had other avenues of escape, before this running away. Her family had wanted her to marry an older man who was economically secure, but she had rejected this culturally approved behavior as personally intolerable. She had tried to become a nun, but the religious life had proven too rigorous for her immaturity and probably the choice had not been adequately enough motivated. In the convent she was lonely and homesick, even for her "bad" home, and was allowed to terminate her period of religious preparation.

The worker saw the challenge that Maria offered: "Could I help her reject and outgrow the undesirable aspects (of her culture) and yet retain and integrate the good factors of her own culture while adapting herself to ours?" It might be queried on theoretic value grounds if a more suitable alternative would not have been to help her develop such personal strengths as were required to adjust in her own culture but unquestionably the destructive reality situation mitigated against this possibility.

At any rate a beauty shop, a teeth-straightening job, new clothes, and a good position found her well on her road to escape. However, things were not entirely that easy.

Maria's relations with men were a problem; she purported to hate them and considered herself at eighteen a hopeless "old maid." A young man at her office "teased" her and made smutty remarks; another asked for a date, whereupon Maria asked him to go to a lecture and he "departed hastily." Her attitudes toward men were hostile and frightened but she responded well to help in understanding these attitudes.

She finally decided to join the WAC. At first I questioned the wisdom of this decision but later realized that the Army would provide a protective, authoritarian atmosphere to which she was accustomed, would fill her need to belong, and would help her with the continuing process of becoming an American.

Throughout these case records there are many references to problems that seem to grow out of conflicts between the client's "culture" and that of the worker. This is hardly surprising; a moment's reflection would tell us that it is almost inevitable. Any helping effort that is centered on the relationship between two people must involve them *as people* and hence as the bearers of certain standards, goals, values, etc., which may not always be in agreement. "Objectivity" in such relationships represents at best an ideal to be sought; it should never be assumed to preclude the inevitable differences between people.[19]

For example: a client seeks help at a Travelers Aid Society for a whole array of problems growing out of severe, chronic, and unmanageable alcoholism. The only noteworthy thing about the client is, in a sense, his "averageness": the spoiled son and brother of a relatively secure and stable family; many efforts at education, jobs, opportunities for "fresh starts" all invariably ruined by his alcoholism; the swings between bravado and contriteness; the inevitable plea for another chance; the rapid shift in behavior and attitudes when sober. The worker says: "When I saw Mr. R. today I was frankly a little surprised to find him sober. With some show of humor, he remarked that I was probably surprised to find that he came back at all and then not dead drunk. I admitted that I had considered that as a possibility, but was glad it had worked out that way." Anyone who has ever tried to help an alcoholic will know exactly how the worker felt! Especially when we find in the record that two days later "Mr. R. came to the booth today, very drunk."

The vagaries of this particular client are not our concern here and I don't want to get involved in a discussion of the larger problem of the etiology, dynamics, and management of alcoholism, as important as these undoubtedly are, especially in an agency like Travelers Aid where alcoholic clients apparently come for help in sizable numbers.

Let us rather look at the worker's evaluation of this case:

While we have no information concerning Mr. Robertson's childhood, it would seem from his present behavior that there was emotional deprivation and possible rejection by those whom he loved.

It is apparent from the note written by his brother that he has little understanding of his real feelings and emotional needs. He asked that I give him a good talking-to for him. Mr. Robertson's aunt and uncle probably follow the same pattern of remonstrance, accusation, and cajolery.

I think that I might have planned with them to help Mr. Robertson go to New Orleans to secure, if possible, a berth on a ship. He might have been able to obtain work, having demonstrated that he does not need alcohol for protracted periods (as when in jail). It is possible that he could have worked again. I should have discussed this at length with Mr. Robertson, learning more about his past experience in the merchant marine and the real possibility of reemployment. It might have been possible for the Travelers Aid worker in New Orleans to meet Mr. Robertson upon his arrival there and to give him sufficient support until he could ship out. This plan would have been in lieu of psychiatric help which Mr. Robertson was not ready or able to use at this time, but might come to later since he apparently is an intelligent person.

I recognize my prejudice toward alcoholism and alcoholics is based on my cultural background and rigid Methodist rearing in a protected environment in a very small town. Also it has a deeper meaning for me, as one member of the family caused us as much anguish as did Mr. Robertson his relatives. This, I think, accounted also for my rejection of Mr. Robertson to the point where I was blocked in using any skill toward helping him establish a truly meaningful relationship with me as a mother person. If I had done this, I might have enabled him to realize his feelings of anxiety and rejection and some of the guilt in his hostility. This might have led to his acceptance of psychiatric help. I realize that I learned little about his problem, as to whether he is an alcoholic, or a problem drinker, etc. If it eventuated in Mr. Robertson returning to the home of his aunt and uncle in Memphis for psychiatric help, a casework agency in that community might have been successful in drawing the aunt and uncle into casework counseling in relation to Mr. Robertson and his problem.

As it is, I feel that Mr. Robertson will continue his present pattern of behaviour until someone helps him utilize his intelligence and his strength.

It is obviously important that the worker realize so clearly the nature and, at least in part, the origins of her own attitudes toward alcoholism. What I found most disturbing in this evaluation was the excessive (to me) sense of failure and guilt. Undoubtedly my own evaluation of this situation is colored by my long experience in the treatment of alcoholics and my almost complete failure with them as a group. I know there are psychiatrists and psychoanalysts who speak glowingly of their results with alcoholics; I can only confess that my own experience is to the contrary and I have seen many of the supposedly "cured" when they have subsequently "relapsed." I felt that this worker was unduly severe in her estimate of the potentialities in the treatment of this man and almost naïvely optimistic about what might have been done "IF"—including "psychiatric referral," that *ultima thule* of the caseworker.

I have said elsewhere [20] that the personality which the social worker brings to his job is a complex resultant of many forces and that in the development of this personality, cultural forces have played a vital role:

That his attitudes towards himself, his clients and his job reflect his own life experiences, his values and goals, his expectancies and ambitions, and his image of himself as a person in a social setting; that these experiences will reflect not only the worker's racial, economic, and religious background and upbringing but also his social class status and that of his family, his class allegiances and awareness and especially in our country, practices and habits of thought and behavior which are native to the particular region in which he spent his formative years; and that these attitudes and goals and needs may conflict with those of his clients who are also materially influenced by their own culture; and that even when there is no conflict, the worker's own culturally influenced attitudes must inevitably play an important role in his understanding, handling, and treatment of the client's problems and, finally, that this interaction is not by any means always conscious and recognized but often, as with other human attitudes, may be active entirely at an unconscious level, disguised in rationalization, and rationalized in theoretical assumptions and technical procedures.

The inordinate length of this sentence aside, I had intended it to convey something of the breadth and depth of these interrelations and, indirectly, to emphasize the all-inclusiveness of the culture concept and the vastly complicated and difficult problems which the acceptance of this concept surely sets up for social workers, as well as others who try to help people. I believe such factors can intrude into the client-worker relationship and make it impossible for a given worker to do a fruitful job with a particular client because of conflicts stemming from cultural differences. But professional understanding should at least minimize the assumption of guilt and self-blame when it is recognized, as in this instance, that a conflict does exist and spare the worker any need to define what seems to me fairly perfectionist attitudes and goals for himself.

To take another case in which this general problem is raised: A woman consulted the Travelers Aid Society for help in obtaining custody of her son who was at that time "boarding" with his maternal grandparents. The client, an American woman of Italian parentage, had married out of her religion, which upset her family very much. This marriage was a failure and ended in divorce. This, too, had created great tensions in her relationship with her Catholic family; the client responded to a question by the worker, "We wondered if Mrs. S. had really renounced the Catholic faith?" by saying "that she had not withdrawn from the church, but that she didn't go any more and that she just could not accept it." She had remarried and her second husband was hospitalized for tuberculosis. The issue between her mother and herself, nominally around the residence of the child, obviously reflected much more deeply rooted conflicts about religion, child-parent-grandparent competition, rejection and guilt, etc.

An evaluation attached to the record states: "Worker was not warm and accepting of Mrs. S. so that the latter could feel that the worker would or could help her with her problems. Worker was struggling with the environmental planning as she saw it and not relating to Mrs. S.'s cultural pattern and great need for emotional support at this time." I would think it an intrusion to comment on the casework aspects of this case (although I must at least say I find no evidence of such inadequacies in the record) but I am constrained to ask just what is meant by the remark "not relating to Mrs. S.'s cultural pattern." The record, understandably, does not offer data sufficient to make definitive statements about this case but such cultural factors as are apparent seem in this instance to be secondary to serious personality distortions. Although it is surely a matter of great moment when a person, especially a Catholic, renounces his religion and marries out of his faith, the roots of such behavior are usually if not always to be found in serious inter- and intra-personal conflict.

I believe that to have expected a caseworker to deal with such factors, disguised as failures in a "cultural pattern," distorts the meaning and value of the more suitable use of cultural concepts. The cultural conflicts of Italian vs. American, Catholic vs. non-Catholic, urban living vs. rural living, seem to me in this case to be rather the backdrop against which the emotional problems are displayed: i.e., hostility and rejection of parents, marital discord and failure, the surrender of the child to the mother's parents at a time of panic and flight, markedly ambivalent attitudes toward the child, etc. I would be concerned about any notion that such a degree of emotional illness can be dealt with primarily in cultural terms, although I recognize the importance of the worker's recognition that such factors exist.

Often in the records one finds such a statement as this one, taken from the record of a 26-year-old Philippine student who went into considerable and quite disproportionate panic when she was not met at the station as had been planned: "Worker was unfamiliar with Philippine cultural patterns and was unable to determine whether the fears expressed were due to environmental background or whether this girl was extremely diffident and possibly emotionally disturbed."

In the first place, I think we should agree that especially in any agency like the Travelers Aid Society it is manifestly impossible for any worker conceivably to be familiar with the cultural patterns of all her clients. In my small sampling of the records they range from American Indian to gypsy and over as widely dispersed a group of cultures and subcultures as one can conceive. It is reasonable to expect that a worker recognize that cultural factors play a role, and perhaps in a given agency dealing with large numbers of a particular subgroup that he familiarize himself with the customs and practices of that group. To expect much beyond that would seem to me to be sheer perfectionism.

A corollary to this general question is raised by a consideration of the suitability of assigning a worker of a given racial group to treat others of the same or other groups. This problem emerges most clearly in connection with the role of the Negro worker.

Several records bear such notations as "in it we have both the Puerto Rican and Negro factors with a Negro worker handling the situation." Or, "this situation was also handled by a Negro worker," in this instance referring to a white client. Or, "this case was handled by a Negro worker and we feel was interesting because of the fact that the client was able to discuss his feeling of racial discrimination quite freely."

This last case is especially apposite and I should like to consider it fairly fully before discussing the general subject of the role of the Negro worker.

Mr. D., a psychiatric attendant, came to the Travelers Aid Society seeking help with employment in a strange city in which he was stranded. The client was a pretentious, boastful man who, the worker said, "had delusions of grandeur." She goes on to say: "Questioned man about hospital experience, as one might assume that he is post-psychiatric." He flatly refused to work in any "non-segregated" hospital. He had, indeed, at the time of his appeal for help from the Travelers Aid Society already refused suitable and gainful work in several hospitals simply because they were non-segregated. He wanted to work in a hospital where "they were all white patients and no Jewish people or Negroes."

The worker discussed job realities with him and then adds:

We discussed his feeling of racial discrimination. I said that he had a perfect right to his own feelings but that I thought he should consider whether or not his personal feelings were being a handicap to him in being able to get a job and support himself. He seemed to have no feeling that I was a Negro person and, I felt, related very well after coming in to the interview. He mentioned that he had no feelings personally against Negroes or Jewish people but that he just never had had contact with them and he did not see why he should begin now. He had been reared in the south where there was a pattern of segregation and he supposed this pattern had remained with him. . . . He seemed to gain some satisfaction out of my acceptance of his feeling of racial discrimination and in relation to me seemed not to have any feeling whatever of talking to me. Finally, necessity compelled him to take a job in a non-segregated hospital; he had decided "it was more important for him to eat than to feel!"

The worker commented: "I said I thought that this was important and that, also, feelings were important, too, in the kind of adjustment a person makes to a job."

I have had no personal experience in working in a clinic or hospital with Negro social workers but I am quite clear on personal and theoretical grounds as to where I stand. A worker should be engaged and his services utilized without any regard to his race, creed, or color or that of the clients. I am, of course, not so naïve as to believe that this is practiced even in those social agencies to which one theoretically should look for enlightenment and advanced attitudes. I know of an agency in New York City where Negro workers are assigned only Negro families as clients with the pathetically patent rationalization that a Negro worker seen on a public vehicle with a white child might be mistaken for a "domestic," to the worker's embarrassment. And I know of still another agency where, despite great to-do about the acceptance of clients without regard to race or creed, a Negro may not be employed even in a secretarial role by fiat of the board.

Since my personal conviction is based largely on feeling rather than experience I decided to find out what others have said or written on this subject. The literature is modest but I found it highly informative. Perhaps the most helpful article I saw was by Luna Brown, called "Race as a Factor in Establishing a Casework Relationship." [21] I think it suitable to review this in some detail.

This paper reports the results of a survey of the situation in social agencies in thirteen states of the northwest. Two hundred fifty-three Negro caseworkers were carrying *un-*

differentiated caseloads; some with only a few, others with a majority of white clients. Eighty per cent of the agencies reported that they had no difficulty whatsoever because of this factor; twenty per cent reported that there had been serious difficulties with Negro workers and white clients. The definition of "serious" is obviously purely relative and difficult to define in this context. As a psychotherapist I know that every therapeutic relationship encounters serious difficulties from time to time; that, in fact, we expect a patient to be able to work out just such hostile and negative feelings in the therapy almost as a prerequisite for getting well. Such attitudes frequently are expressed around the therapist's religion or race, as indeed they may be about almost anything else. I am always interested to note that when summer comes and I begin to wear bow ties at least one or two patients will express feelings of ridicule, resentment, or distaste about them. I realize that the casework relationship ordinarily does not permit the exploration and understanding of complicated transference realtionships but I think that anyone trying to understand this problem would think twice before accepting, as fact, a client's statement as to the source of the difficulty in a relationship. And I would caution against looking for the "cure" of the difficulty in abolishing the so-called "cause." If one is not careful in understanding that the tensions attributed to the difference in race may actually be only rationalizations or projections of deeper unconscious hostility, one might arrive at the dubious solution of "matching" worker and client.[22]

Despite the fairly large proportion (20 per cent) of agencies that reported difficulty, *only one* agency thought it unwise for Negro workers to carry white clients, and there were very few reported instances where an agency found it necessary to transfer a client. (I could find no comparable data on the frequency with which such transfer is necessary in ordinary agency practice for other reasons. I would imagine it must not be at all unusual.) One agency commented: "If a client, Negro or white, shows resistance to using or accepting the caseworker because of race, the matter is discussed with the client insofar as is compatible with understanding the resistance, yet stopping short of imposing on a client an additional hurdle to using our service." Unfortunately I lack the experience and knowledge which would entitle me to an opinion about a statement like that and I realize it is not reasonable to make parallels with private psychiatric practice. Frankly, I must say that this seems too timid a concept. However, I realize that a purely pragmatic attitude may well justify it.

Some of the Negro workers reported that some Negro clients preferred workers of their own race, others felt insecure and looked on a Negro worker as inadequate and inferior. Basically, such attitudes reflect one's feelings about oneself; if a person equates his being a Negro with being inadequate, inferior, "dirty," etc., he will automatically project such attitudes on to his Negro worker. This identical pattern of thinking and feeling is often encountered among members of other minority groups. Similarly a Negro who consciously or unconsciously resents being a Negro and is trying to "escape" will reject a Negro worker. Here again such attitudes are commonly found among other minority groups.

Miss Brown mentions other attitudes which proved intrusive in the relationship between Negro worker and client. Some of these, understandably, were found in the workers themselves. The inexperienced or insecure Negro worker, afraid of rejection by his white colleagues, might prove overdemanding toward white clients or, on occasion, too permissive. Such a worker might well deny his feelings against Negro clients but actually demand more of them by way of conformity and adequacy of performance, often judging this by the most conventional "white" mores. Negro clients often sense this and prefer white workers who are apt to be less demanding. Of course, some of these white workers are less demanding of high standards of compliance and achievement in Negro clients because of their (the workers') own culturally imposed estimate of the Negro's capacities and potentialities, or perhaps because of some unconscious desire to keep them "second-class" citizens.

In any discussion such as this we must be careful to distinguish, insofar as that is possible, between culturally determined patterns and those actually foisted on people by poverty and its almost inevitable concomitants of ignorance, inadequate health standards, poor housing, and the evils attendant on it, etc. I know that I have made this point before but it is worth repeating; unless we bear these distinctions in mind we leave ourselves open to the confusion that leads directly to stereotyping on which prejudicial attitudes flourish.

This distinction is underscored in several of our cases. A family of American migrant fruit pickers sought help. This family illustrates all the usual facets of poverty—the whole family, for instance, sleeps in one room, parents and four children, three boys, 14, 10, and 8 and a girl of four, the latter in her parents' bed; the children's education has been haphazard and they are all "back" in their grades; John, the eldest, is only in sixth grade at 14 and Dickie, aged 10, is said to be "sub-normal"; they have chronic malnutrition and are generally deprived. Any comment on the emotional impact of this hand-to-mouth existence would be superfluous. The mother tells, for instance, that she feels quite safe in leaving the children in what even she considers an undesirable neighborhood "since they have been trained to fear 'winos,' have come up against lots of 'winos' in the family's traveling." When they see a "wino" coming they hide because she has warned them: "They'll kill you!" On Halloween the children were too scared to go out for very long and came running back into the house after just a few minutes although it was still light out. "Mrs. O. seemed to think that this was good training and that they should be fearful and stay close to home in this way."

There are several clients who come from groups who are seriously handicapped because of prevalent and widely believed stereotypes. Besides the Negroes and the Jews, the Armenians, the gypsies, and the Puerto Ricans all represent such manifestations of prejudiced stereotyping.

This matter of stereotyping is of the greatest importance. It is the substance on which prejudice fattens, and entails exactly the sort of prejudgment which the word "prejudice" describes. As long as we say the Armenians never pay their bills, the Jews care only for money, the Negroes all eat too many pork chops and spend their time gambling and carousing, we have made it impossible to understand adequately the *individual* with whom we are concerned, in whatever the relationship.

A few comments on the dynamics of prejudice may be in order at this point.

Prejudice is a highly complicated phenomenon, known throughout much of the history of the human race. It has been extensively studied and discussed but is by no means as yet adequately understood. It has been defined as a "pattern of hostility in interpersonal relations which is directed against an entire group or against its individual members; it fulfills a specific irrational function for the bearer." [23] To try to think of it in basically psychodynamic terms risks some distortion of our understanding of the phenomenon, since the very question implies that prejudice is ultimately to be understood in terms of the personality. To be sure, insofar as prejudice is expressed by people and groups and directed against other people and groups, the dynamic factors are of great moment but beyond these we must try to understand prejudice as a phenomenon which has social, economic, cultural, and religious factors involved in its causation and expression, and which requires a sound historical basis for its understanding. Thus, while it can be said that prejudice is endemic in the world, there have been over the centuries acute and virulent "epidemics," as at the time of the Inquisition, or more recently under the Hitler terror. Although it is interesting and important, for instance, to try to understand the personality of Hitler,[24] it is naïve to assume that even the fullest understanding of the man, his genesis and "sickness" could explain the historical phenomena of Nazi Germany. As Fenichel said:

The psychoanalysis of anti-Semites is indispensable if anti-Semitism is to be understood. But it is in no way sufficient to explain it. After a study of the influences determining the structure of the anti-Semitic personality and of how this structure functions, the question of the genesis of these influences and of the social function of the anti-Semitic reaction still remains unanswered.[25]

The psychological and psychoanalytic studies of prejudice are numerous and the literature continues to grow. Perhaps the best known of these works is the series of studies [26] done under the aegis of the American Jewish Committee. One of the basic insights gained from these studies is a concept of the personality distortion which leads to authoritarian attitudes and prejudicial behavior. This personality, as described by Brunswik, tends to be a restricted, narrow personality with a strict conventional super-ego, to which there is complete surrender. It is the conventional super-ego which takes over the function of the underdeveloped ego, producing a lack of individualism and a tendency to stereotyped thinking. In order to achieve harmony with parents, the parental images and with society as a whole, basic impulses which are conceived of as low, destructive and dangerous have to be kept repressed and can find only devious expressions, as for instance, in projections and "moral indignation." Thus, anti-Semitism and intolerance against out-groups generally may have an important function in keeping the personality integrated. Without these channels or outlets (if they should not be provided by society) it may be much more difficult, in some cases impossible, to keep the mental balance. Hence, the rigid and compulsive adherence to prejudices.[27]

A number of highly significant statements may be made on the basis of the psychoanalytic studies of prejudice. Anti-Semitism [28] is not the concomitant of any one clinical category of personality disturbance. The absence of true depressions in the Ackerman and Jahoda cases is particularly striking and significant. The existence of the prejudiced attitude "presupposes a tendency to blame the outside world rather than one's own self, and, dynamically, such a tendency is in contradiction to the self-destructive features of a genuine depression." [29]

Certain emotional predispositions to anti-Semitism can be isolated. These character tendencies and reactions are not in themselves specific in the causation of anti-Semitism and they can exist without anti-Semitism. However, this and probably other forms of prejudice do not exist without such disturbances in the personality. First among these is anxiety, usually quite pervasive and manifesting itself indirectly in various forms of social discomfort and disability. "Socially, economically, emotionally and sexually they are plagued by (an) exaggerated sense of vulnerability." [30] These people view the outside world as "hostile, evil and inexplicably hard."

A second characteristic is the confusion of the concept of self. As Ackerman and Jahoda state:

So confused and vague is their self-image that they do not seem to know who or what they are, what they desire and what they can forego . . . with little regard for facts and the external situation of their lives they waver between feelings of inferiority and superiority; between regarding themselves as strong or weak, and between considering themselves as members of this or that group, or as completely isolated human beings.[31]

A third point which should be emphasized is the fact that the prejudiced person, because of an unstable and confused self-image, is unable to achieve satisfactory interpersonal relations. This absence of warm human relations causes these people shame and suffering and leads them to great emphasis on a shallow conformity to group standards.

It is not surprising to learn that these people lack a consistent value system protected by a well-developed conscience. Hence, they do not feel guilty about their prejudiced attitudes and behavior.

Of consequence in the genesis of such prejudiced attitudes are poor relationships between parents, quarreling, divorce, and the other familiar manifestations of such failures in marriage. One or both parents were usually rejecting of the child and there are serious unresolved oedipal conflicts in the prejudiced persons.

Further insight into the anti-Semitic attitudes emphasizes the extent to which such people use their prejudice as "a profound though irrational and futile defensive effort to restore a crippled self [and] at the social level . . . as a device for achieving secondary emotional and material gain." [32] To examine the data on which such statements are made would lead us far astray; I can only recommend a serious perusal of at least some of the relevant literature.

There are, of course, other ideas about prejudice than those contained in psychoanalytic theory. It has been likened, for instance, to a conditioned reflex; as Murphy describes this aspect of the subject:

When we say, "I dislike Jones and I really don't know why; I suppose I'm just prejudiced," this represents a kind of response which may well be due to one disagreeable incident in the past or even to an incident which did not concern Jones himself at all but someone who looked like him. It may be that in early childhood we were caught red-handed and given a good shaking by someone who shared some superficial physical attribute with the Jones of today, something like a mustache or stooped shoulders or a long nose.

Murphy goes on to say:

It must be granted that this simpler type of carry-over from an earlier sharp experience does occasionally play *some* (author's italics) part in the phenomenon of prejudice. [33]

There are undoubtedly group or cultural factors which at least contribute toward instilling prejudice; after all, children imitate parents and parent surrogates in matters of attitudes and preferences as well as in their behavior, and many a child says he "hates" some thing or person or group or "loves" another long before he has had any experience with the thing or persons involved. There are regions of the country where certain prejudices are almost universal, such as the anti-Catholic feelings in certain districts of the southeastern part of the country. In general, we trust "our own kind" and equate our own with the good and acceptable; those who are outside the group are viewed with caution and doubt, even, at times of hardship, with actual hostility. It requires a sound and secure youngster to learn to accept the "others" as his peers and not to project on to them his failures and defeats. Children easily separate into "we" and "they," the safe and the threatening, the "rights" and the "wrongs."

It is in this connection that economic competition comes to play so basic a role in prejudice. Where a group is secure and not in any way threatened by economic competition from an out-group, its tolerance is infinitely greater than where the out-group is or seems to be a threat to the economic life of the group. This accounts for the familiar increase in prejudice and outbreaks of hostility in times of depression and social tension.

Here we must recognize that the threat to economic security may in fact be nonexistent, often merely the projection of pre-existing hostility and prejudice. For instance, the Jews are said "to control the banks, the department stores, the motion-picture industry, etc." This is believed to be true despite all the evidence [34] to the contrary and is then exploited as a justification for anti-Semitism. It is obviously not the facts that make the prejudice but the prejudice that distorts and exaggerates the "facts."

Murphy points out another influence making for prejudice which he terms "interference and exclusion." He says:

It may happen that those who do not share our values actually *interfere* (italics in the original) in a direct and obvious way with our pursuit of our own values. This will ordinarily not occur on a large scale under conditions which Americans encounter in the matter of religious affiliation. The worship on Sunday morning in many different churches need not involve any opposition, resistance, vituperation by one group with reference to another. They are simply separate groups worshiping in their separate houses of worship. But let the issue be defined, however, in such a way that the pursuit of what is good, necessary, and valuable by one group *interferes* (italics in the original) with the similar pursuit of what is good, necessary, and valuable by another group. Take such a very simple illustration as the marked reduction in the number of jobs that can be filled or the area which can be cultivated as a result of such a social catastrophe as a storm damaging the factories and business district of a city or a flood making most of the land incapable of cultivation. Now ill feeling is likely to arise immediately if it turns out that the availability of jobs or of land depends in any way upon group membership. If, for example, there is a lively organization of the Baptists which gets jobs for its boys under this condition of crisis, it is likely that the Catholics, the Methodists, the Jews, in effect every non-Baptist, will express (along with admiration for the go-getting qualities of the Baptists) a certain amount of hostility for the unfairness of the whole operation. In the same way, if a politically astute leader manages to get boats and farm implements quickly to the region of the land which is capable of cultivation so that only those of a particular political party have land which they can cultivate before too late in the season, there is likely to be intense feeling on the part of other political groups that a march has been stolen upon them.

We have begun with relatively trivial illustrations. Let us expand this until we have the scene in which only the members of one religious, racial, or ethnic group can obtain special favors or privileges, particularly such as admission to educational institutions or admission to apprenticeships which give them in course of time desirable skilled trades to practice. This kind of exclusiveness does exist all over the civilized world to some extent, and alert groups who care something about democracy are forever fighting such issues; e.g., issues as to whether Jews are to be kept out of certain clubs or Negroes out of certain universities. "Social tension" is obviously present on both sides of the coin, on the side of those who try to break in and on the side of those who try to keep them out.[35]

He points out that such local or temporary circumstances are apt to be generalized and then set in rigid prejudiced attitudes and feeling. From such attitudes it is just a short step to the stereotype, that fixed attitude which is so difficult to correct.

Another serious aspect of this tendency to stereotype people is that the stereotype tends to perpetuate itself. Thus, if the Negro is believed to be shiftless, this very attitude makes it difficult for him to get steady work and abets his shiftlessness if indeed it ever existed.

There are other sources of prejudice, such as unconscious feelings of hostility which may be projected on to a person or group who are conceived, often irrationally, as obstacles toward the goals the individual cherishes. Then there are the projections of our own feelings of inadequacy and failure, of guilt and hostility, on to others who represent the very things against which the individual is unconsciously struggling. Both of these aspects of prejudice have been thoroughly investigated psychoanalytically.[36]

Prejudice is a complicated subject indeed and I have done little more than touch on some of its aspects. Fortunately, the literature is rich and varied and readily available for the interested reader.[37]

To return to the Travelers Aid cases, the various points already made are further illustrated in a number of cases of which I shall mention a few. The danger of stereotyping is effectively demonstrated in the instance of an aggressive, self-seeking, ambitious woman who seemed to fit the worker's (and the usual American) concept of a "German," but who actually was an Austrian. If there is validity in the concept of "national character" she is typically of the German category, not an easy-going, relaxed, unaggressive Austrian. At any rate what seems more important in this case than the label is the worker's understanding of this woman's need to try to compensate for her own lacks (illegitimacy, childhood deprivations, etc.) by "success" and by providing for her own children the very things she had lacked, especially security and a "strong (good) father." This is a dynamic which would seem surely to cut across national boundaries.

Two cases of gypsy women present a number of important questions. The first case is that of a woman in her middle 30's who sought help for her four children and herself. She was determined to get them all on a particular train and demanded that the Travelers Aid Society supply the necessary funds. They were bedraggled, dirty, frightened, and weary. The entire family had been traveling with a carnival and her husband had left, presumably to secure more remunerative employment. She had not heard from him in several weeks and had been chasing over the country trying to track him down in response to one or another rumor as to his whereabouts. She had considered herself divorced under gypsy law for the past three months because of nonsupport, although she had apparently been living with him until two weeks previously. She was now trying to return to New York where her father and brothers lived and were on relief. The distracted woman refused all offers of help other than the one she demanded and was last seen trying to board the train of her choice.

In this instance, the elements of cultural influence seem secondary to a serious and damaging personality disorder, although there is hardly enough data to warrant much speculation about its nature. She seems to be a dependent, "psychopathic" person, planless and irresponsible and too disturbed to accept help.

In the second so-called gypsy case (she was actually of Russian extraction but her family was considered gypsy) we are dealing with a very disturbed woman whose husband had deserted her with another woman and taken four of their five children, their trailer in which they traveled with carnivals, and the money that she had hidden in the trailer.

This case illustrates only too well how difficult it is to separate cultural from personality elements and seriously raises the question of how necessary it is for a worker dealing, as here, with a reality problem to "understand the culture" of the client. Obviously, if one were involved in a therapeutic effort designed to alter the client's basic personality structure the need to understand such cultural (genetic) factors would surely be greater. I raise this question especially since a note attached to the record states: "In this situation, our worker felt completely stymied because of lack of understanding of the gypsy cultural background. . . ."

Actually, there were some confusing elements in this situation related to gypsy customs. For instance, the client was in mortal dread of retribution because she had committed two "sins." She had resorted to American rather than gypsy law in an effort to have her husband apprehended and punished and secondly she had cursed her mother-in-law, which is said to have special meaning to gypsies but which the client said she could not explain.

There were undoubtedly these cultural elements but I felt from reading the record that the client was behaving like many other wives whose husbands have deserted with other women and who find themselves stranded, without resources, frightened and confused. Her markedly ambivalent attitudes toward her husband are not at all unique; I am sure she wanted both to see him punished and to think of him as returning, contrite, and once more loving and devoted. The pathology in this case is of an order which is difficult to evaluate and it undoubtedly presents factors derived from her cultural background. If we assume a continuum of external (environmental) and internal factors influencing the individual's character and personality structure, it cannot be otherwise. However where, as in this situation, the challenge is to help the individual with the immediate reality situation and not, as perhaps in other therapeutic relationships, with a revision of the personality, I feel that the emphasis on "failure" is unwarranted as is the apparent need to understand the client's "culture" in every instance.

I would like to mention one more case. A note on a worker's visit to a lower middle-class Chinese home in a southern industrial city states that the family was lacking in all "cultural opportunities." I gather that what the worker meant is that they lacked a TV set, didn't go to movies, etc. It seems highly unlikely from the description of the family and their desire to have their child educated in a Chinese school, etc., that they lacked *Chinese* cultural opportunities.

I have tried to define culture in such a way as to emphasize its part in the development of the individual and its influence on the personality and character structure. I have used the case material essentially to highlight the importance for all of us who work with people of having a genuine awareness of the meaning of culture and of its impact on the development and current life situation of the person we are serving. I have tried to emphasize, too, the importance of the worker's own culture and to illustrate the extent to which a person's own attitudes and bias may intrude into the casework relationship.

Throughout the discussion I have tried to point out the significance of the concept of culture in social work while trying to keep it in the proper focus and in some measure to warn against what I consider the risks inherent in the overemphasis of the concept for social caseworkers, among others. To appreciate fully the importance of a point of view is not to attribute everything to it or to make it more than it is, in this instance a mighty tool for understanding and helping people in trouble.

8. WHAT UNEMPLOYMENT
DOES TO PEOPLE

PSYCHIATRY, so long fettered to the insane asylum and pre-occupied with the problems of disease and its alleviation, has only recently ventured to put its skills and techniques at the service of those concerned with the human being in his "normal" interests and ways of life. Cautiously, and rightly so, the psychiatrist has joined with the sociologist, the criminologist, the economist to explore fields of mutual interest and to attempt thus to study the human being in settings and faced with problems and tasks not uniquely involved in the questions of disease.[1]

Psychiatry, itself a new discipline in the family of the sciences, has felt that it must surround itself with every safeguard in these trial testings of its knowledge in the borderline fields of human enterprise. The immediate application of the knowledge of individual behavior to that of the group by multiplication, as it were, is a thoroughly dangerous one that has led to much confusion and even to some nonsense. However it is certain that cautiously and tentatively applied, psychiatric insights can illuminate many human problems and at the same time, enrich its own more immediate spheres of interest.

Consider, for example, the lack of opportunity the psychiatrist and even the psychoanalyst has for the study of relatively normal, average people. Inevitably, the study of the sick person is enhanced by knowledge of people free of serious pathology. Only in the collaborative efforts of social scientist and psychiatrist can such experience be obtained.

Psychiatrists are constantly beset with the need more adequately to estimate the setting in which disease occurs; to evaluate factors of daily routine and adjustment antedating the apparent development of mental disease. A most important part of this world, it seemed to us, was the work a man did, the rewards it afforded him, and his adjustments to the loss of work.

But perhaps even more in the field of the neuroses knowledge about the work-a-day world seemed scant and we hoped to learn substantially more about it. The neurotic is almost characteristically unhappy on his job or unable to keep one; disorganized in his quest for advancement and suitable enterprise. The phrase "neurotic work history" has become a commonplace. The psychotherapist, often called on to estimate the patient's own estimate of his job, his desires to "quit" and the rationalizations for this desire, and analogous problems, could perhaps, if only in a peripheral sense, also profit from studies of this sort.

This report summarizes some of the findings of an interdisciplinary effort to study the impact of unemployment on a carefully selected group of families in New York City at the end of the great depression of the 1930s. In brief, it is a report on what unemployment does to people.

Since unemployment entailed for some, loss of work and income and for others only loss of income, part of the sample was drawn from the Home Relief rolls (financial aid without work); the other from WPA (work relief). Three groups were chosen; Irish-Catholics, Jews, and Anglo-Saxon Protestants, to test whether racial-cultural factors influenced adjustment to unemployment. It was believed, for instance, that to get any clear picture of what unemployment did to the Negro would require a comprehensive study of the adjustment of the Negro in community life— itself a vastly complex problem. We also excluded from the sample those families in which the head of the household was over fifty-five at the time of the study or severely handicapped for reemployment for physical or psychological reasons. The importance of this limitation is primary since to have included heads of families already known to be handicapped by emotional or mental illness would have invalidated our purpose: to study the effect of unemployment on "normal" people.

We are thoroughly aware of the risks involved in the use of such an ill defined term as "normal." We felt relatively safe however in including as normal those who had shown no overt signs of mental or emotional difficulty, who after some years of privation and hardship had not broken down into neurotic illness or deviant behavior. We also believed that the establishment of the requirement of whole families would tend to insure a certain basic adequacy, viewing divorce more often than not as an indication of emotional tensions within the family.

Included in the sample was a control group, in part composed of families who had previously been on relief but were now again self-supporting and in part of families of low income but who had never been on relief. Without this control group it would have been impossible to know whether our findings about the families on relief were truly the result of unemployment or were rather the result of other trends in the economy and the culture.

Two hundred and fifty families in all were studied, but the final sample consisted of 180 families. The data in the records of these families in the District Offices of the Department of Welfare, WPA, and N.Y. State Employment Service were carefully abstracted, and our staff subsequently had an opportunity to discuss each family with the Home Relief investigator or case supervisor to whom it was known. Social workers visited every family at home and had long interviews with the women and frequently the men. Incidentally, it ought to be mentioned that initial cooperation was obtained in all but one Home Relief and two WPA cases as the result of a simple letter setting forth our plan to study the problem of unemployment and requesting their cooperation, but in no way promising or suggesting any sort of reward.

In retrospect I have thought that this extraordinary response on the part of people of the most limited education and background was already a suggestion of their substantial integration, which the study was abundantly to confirm. At the same time the worker had an opportunity to observe the children and their relationship with their parents and siblings, and to talk with the older children. In addition, many of the men and older children were interviewed by the economist and myself.

We are quite aware of the fact that from a psychiatric point of view our material is entirely superficial, as any data obtained solely by the interview method must inevitably be. However, we think it strictly comparable to other psychiatric material obtained in interviews and much more complete than the material on which the psychiatrist is frequently asked to base an opinion.[2] The amount and accuracy of the material is primarily a tribute to the skills of my social work colleagues.

For years, quite insidiously, we had been sold a concept of the unemployed. No group ever afforded so happy an opportunity for exploitation and derision, or so rich a source for bias and emotional distortion. The abundant WPA jokes, the callous cartoons, the insinuating editorial all reflected and helped create an utterly distorted picture of the unemployed man and his family.

What sort actually were the people who made up our material; whence had they come, what were their interests and ambitions, their sources of comfort and pleasure, their devotions and beliefs, their expectations for their children, and their feelings toward their country.

Almost the first thing we did when we started our study was to clear all the cases through the Social Service Exchange. To our complete surprise no case was known to any welfare or assistance dispensing agency prior to the depression. At first glance this might be construed as a result of their ignorance or failure adequately to use the resources of the community. That this was not the case was demonstrated by their generous, if, to be sure, not always complete use of child health agencies, hospitals and the like. Rather, it proved a substantial piece of evidence of the essential self-sufficiency of these families and of their desire and ability to make a go of it strictly on their own. These were definitely not the chronic "charity" cases, the seekers of communal props for their individual inadequacies.

How had these people, whom the public had been asked to consider bums and failures, come to their plight originally? Only in 4 cases in the Home Relief sample did the men lose their jobs because of personal inadequacies which might be construed as blameworthy—the reason in the case of these four was drinking, to a psychiatrist surely itself a "sickness." Sixty per cent lost their jobs because of reduction in employment or their employers' bankruptcy; 15 per cent because of organic illness. In the WPA group, all but

8 lost their jobs because of the failure or decline of the business in which they were employed; only 2 because of illness and 6 for reasons for which they could in an ethical sense be thought responsible. Four of these 6 were discharged because of drinking. In the group formerly on relief who returned to private employment 27 of 30 had lost their jobs through the decline in their own or their employers' business. In brief, they were overwhelmingly the victims of the world-wide depression for which they surely bore no responsibility.

Prior to seeking relief, these families had for the most part been self-supporting. Only a very few had not been able to earn enough. Their average salary during the 1920s had been more or less representative of the working population in New York City.

What did these people believe in before they were unemployed? All the Catholics and all but one of the Jews were reared in orthodox homes and the great majority had continued to observe the rituals of their religion. Only about one half of the Protestant families had strong religious affiliations. However, only a few families were without some religious ties.

What of the political faiths of these people? It is important to emphasize the extreme averageness of these families politically. They were, as is consistent in New York City, overwhelmingly Democratic, with a scattering of Republicans and but 2 self-styled Communists.

As an index of their adjustment to reality various data are offered, all emphasizing the stability and integrity of these families before unemployment:

(1) Over two thirds of these families had carried life insurance, both as protection and as savings. Many had both insurance and savings bank accounts, few had neither.

(2) Over one third had shown considerable initiative and ingenuity in seeking and obtaining better paying jobs, or those offering what seemed to be better opportunities.

(3) They evinced a universal desire to have their children better themselves in the world of education and training. There were only 24 children in our study over the legal age for leaving school (17) and 9 of them were in school or college at understandable sacrifices to the parents. This also came out quite vividly in the constantly repeated contention of immigrant parents that they would never want to return to the "old country," not so much for their own as for their children's sakes: education here was free and training available and one might make something of himself.

The emotional implications of unemployment are many and profound. First: what is the import of the very act of being fired and losing one's job? Emotionally, the nearest counterpart to this experience is the loss of love the child suffers from a rejecting parent, especially a child who "has not done anything" to deserve it. In this connection, it will be recalled how few of these men lost their jobs for reasons which by any stretch of usage could be called their "fault." In our community the "boss" is for many men a very real parent (father) substitute—the person who provides him with the means for shelter and food, who protects him from various threats (loan-shark rackets for instance), to whom he can, ideally at least, go for advice and help and who looks after his future security. This was especially so for many of the men who had worked long, arduous years for one employer, to whom as well as to the job they had understandably formed real attachments. Many of these men had worked ten to twenty years at one job. Such loyalties and devotion are not easily severed.

Deprived of "love," the first reaction was essentially one

of fear and bewilderment, combined with optimism, born of wishful thinking and obviously overcompensatory in nature. Where an objective estimate of the situation would have led in most instances to pessimism or at least profound skepticism, these men were almost invariably hopeful. They had worked through the "dizzy 20s" when work was abundant; unemployment was a new experience and one not easy to assay. For example: "Mr. C. went everywhere looking for work; he was sure he'd find something." "Mr. R. made the rounds of all the insurance companies" (he had previously been an insurance agent), "Mr. M. was sure unemployment was a temporary thing and that he soon would be able to locate work." "As far as Mrs. F. can remember, her husband's only reaction was to work harder, searching frantically for new orders."

Some of the families, however, responded to this crisis and the implicit withdrawal of affection and security by fear and panic. They were ashamed and painfully aware of the possibility that they might have to resort to charity. "Mr. and Mrs. G. were greatly disturbed by Mr. G.'s loss of work. They had been so secure in their long established business, they did not know where to turn." "Mrs. B. said that their first and strongest feeling had been one of shame because in their opinion it was a disgrace for a man who had formerly had his own business to admit defeat."

It is defeat that most of these families found in their unemployment: defeat and a threat to their status in the community, their ambitions for themselves (however modest they were and assuredly they were scaled most modestly) and their hopes for their children. But few of them were conscious of such implications, especially early in their unemployment.

They proceeded as fast as they could to curtail their

expenses, to borrow, to cash insurance policies (for these people the use of their insurance policies raised the terrifying threat of pauperization: the loss of burial money and a pauper's grave). It represented a real desire for independence, this willingness to sacrifice this protection, symbolic as well as real; to utilize savings, to draw on other members of the family: in brief, and, in sharp contrast to the popular notion, to do anything but go on relief. Of the 60 men on Home Relief, 17 had been unemployed over six months before first applying for relief and 20 up to six months. Only 13 applied within a month after losing their jobs and these were the families where illness, marginal incomes, etc., had made savings virtually impossible.

They also proceeded to look for work. On the average the men looked constantly—in the face of difficulties almost impossible to imagine. Mr. ——— allowed himself ten cents a day on which to seek work; five cents took him all the way downtown, five cents bought him a bar of chocolate each day on his trek back to the Bronx, a distance of ten to twenty miles each day, rain or shine. Sixteen of these families succeeded in regaining a position of self-support for periods sufficient to permit them to come off relief and 20 succeeded in reducing more or less the Home Relief allowance by their earnings in private employment.

With the loss of job goes the great loss of prestige values, within and without one's home. No matter how humble the job, it had sufficed. In our civilization, work is what man lives by. We work to earn the necessities of life, to secure its comforts, to provide as befits a man for our families. It helps still the feelings of inferiority that unconsciously beset us; it gains us parity with our fellows and the acceptance of the community. It dignifies our daily life, no matter how humble. In it we may expend our aggressive impulses and ward off the profound feelings of insecurity and helpless-

ness. With work man earns more than a stipend: he gains
the right to be master in his home. For the unemployed man,
all this is changed.

Perhaps the most pressing problem is the maintenance of
his position in the home. Quickly the children become
aware, and at an early age, of this change in status. One
youngster flatly challenged his parents' authority, saying
"you didn't take care of me, the relief did." The women are
especially sensitive to this loss of prestige and authority on
the part of the father and accurately sense its detrimental
influence on the growing child. Over and over we found
them trying artificially to pump up "dad" as the authority,
to see to it that he did not lose his father rôle. Mothers encouraged the children to take their homework to father for
help; to look to him for consent or denial of special privileges and otherwise to maintain the position which usually
is the father's.

The baneful effects of this situation on the growing child
needs no emphasis to psychiatrists. Whatever discipline of
psychodynamics we may adopt, we may safely agree on
the necessity for an emotionally respected father ideal for
the mental hygiene of the child.

For the man, life deteriorates into a sodden repetition of
job seeking and lounging about the house. He no longer
meets his fellow on the job and whatever limited cama-
raderie was his, no longer exists. Although the unemployed
tend to congregate geographically in certain neighborhoods,
each tries, if naïvely, to hide his handicap from his neighbors. So great is the feeling of shame for being on relief that
13 families had persisted in hiding their status even after
years on relief, even to the extent of refusing to make use
of surplus commodities which would at once have identified them as relief recipients. Many of the children refused
to eat the hot lunches provided for them in school since

this identified them as "reliefers." One rightly estimates such
behavior as highly inadequate and neurotic; it also measures
the profundity of their shame. "You just aren't people any
more on relief." "I worry all the time someone will find
out; it's such a terrible disgrace." "This feeling of receiving
charity is a bitter pill and makes you feel as if you were
dead." "It is taking something for nothing." The nightly
beer has lost its social value and needs to be taken on the
rare occasions when it can be afforded away from accustomed haunts; the conversation no longer can be about the
job, "prospects," the ball game.

At the start of the investigation the staff put the question
to me: "what avenues of protest and compensatory outlet
did I believe would be available to the unemployed man?" I
postulated four: excessive irritability; political revolt, if but
verbal and either to the right or left and the formation of
protest groups; an increase in aggressive sexual demands;
and deviate behavior of various aggressive types, including
criminal behavior.

As if to illustrate the hazards of such more or less theoretically deduced conclusions,[3] the data did not substantiate
these presumptions, with the possible exception of irritability and even here it was in the wives and not especially in
the unemployed men that this was found.

The body of the unemployed is obviously fertile ground
into which to implant protest against the symbol of authority: the state. To test the fermentation of such processes the
men and women were queried about their politics, their attitudes to the relief set-up and to such organizations as the
Workers' Alliance, etc. Those who see the unemployed as
a breeding ground for left or right wing dissident groups
would find small satisfaction in our material. Only 2 families
read left-wing newspapers, and 2 were active in left-wing
groups. The question will be raised as to how accurate such

information is since a desire to conceal political radicalism would be understandable. We believe that the repeated interviews by various members of the staff and the highly scrutinizing attitudes of the workers of the Department of Public Welfare would have sufficed to reveal such movement had it existed. A more middle-of-the-road, average American group could not be found.

The unemployed man at home found his greatest outlet in taking over as many feminine responsibilities as possible, perhaps in expiation for a sense of guilt, perhaps as one of the very few ways available to him for justifying his existence. The men shopped (bargain hunting at a distance from home can be very important on relief budgets), washed, took care of the youngsters, etc. But largely they slunk about the house trying to keep out from underfoot; to be as little obstruction in their idleness as possible, or "vanished" from the house for as long periods as possible without risking the investigator's "suspicion" that they were working.

Their attitudes to their wives reflected no aggressive overcompensation: here too they were without the capacity to revolt. We found bickering, petty irritation, complaints that the men were so constantly about as to preclude normal management of the home, but little suggestion of aggressive demands by the man.

The only evidence of protest behavior which we found was in the religious behavior of our clients. Of the Catholic families, 5 who had not previously done so practiced birth control, but tried otherwise to remain within the fold, and 3 revolted all the way, disowning entirely all religious observances. Three Jewish families, previously orthodox in their practices, ceased to conform. An estimate of this type of behavior is not easy: economic and other factors complicate the picture immensely.

Of crime there was but one instance and this had its obvious roots in the situation which prevailed before the man had become unemployed. There was no increase in drinking; perhaps, to the contrary some lessening, even in those whose drinking had previously involved them in difficulties.

We found a number of attempts to "cheat" on the investigators in petty ways and I believe this afforded them some slight ego gratification, of the kind a child gets from cheating teacher or pilfering pennies from his mother's purse. In addition some increase in their feelings of security probably resulted; having so little, any additional sum, no matter how trivial, could accomplish this, at least symbolically.

It appears definite that one need not fear "revolt" of the unemployed; perhaps it would be better had they greater capacity for protest. This is a group of quite thoroughly discouraged and defeated people, frightened and confused, and clutching only to hope for their children if not for themselves.

We need not concern ourselves here with the economics of work relief: as a mental hygiene device it is unimpeachable. From the psychiatrist's point of view, the defects in work relief are many: the jobs are too frequently entirely unrelated to a man's previous skills or interests; the incentive of reward for a job well done is too little; the community stigmatization of WPA too great a burden; the disciplines of the job too often lax and partisan. But it at least enables a man to work—to get out of the house in the morning to go to the job, to return, perhaps fortunately tired and grimy, having justified one's existence through one's own efforts and to have again the feeling that one is master in one's home. The pressing need to work is satisfied and, whatever their grumbling, the men acknowledge their gratefulness for this: "Mr. M. likes to work and believes that despite the fact some people take advantage of WPA, the majority of the men want to earn their way." "In the opinion of both

Mr. and Mrs. B. WPA is a wonderful thing in that it has given him a chance to work and not to feel he is receiving charity."

Singer[4] in his monograph *Unemployment and the Unemployed* has emphasized the common routine which work enforces on all people who take part in it.

"They get up at the same hour, they have their meals at the same time and in the same way, they are doing the same sort of job all day long, they develop an interest in the same topics as the other people in the firm, such as the prospects of the trade, wages, working conditions, hours. . . . Their very thoughts, ideas, behavior, way of dressing, the words they use are molded into a common pattern, very often without their knowing it."

This routine vanishes with unemployment; and the freedom from the routine becomes a curse. It is a freedom conditioned by poverty, which limits every activity: "we only listen to the radio at night; the electric bills are too high to listen in the daytime." "Yes, we might visit a friend or relative, but look at our clothes and then they'd expect to visit us and we'd have to offer them something and we haven't any decent dishes any more."

But unemployment is not just a vacuum state, one of mere waiting about for a new job. The day must be filled: men are not beef that can be put in the refrigerator and kept fresh until needed. Attitudes are formed, bitterness and disillusionment fostered, skills lost, self-discipline relaxed, habits of neatness and punctuality and ability to work with one's fellow dissipated. And over all is developed a protective layer of "not-thinking," of refusal to contemplate one's problems or the awfulness of one's plight: an anesthetic to deaden one's pains.

Obviously, this is a most unhealthy mental state, for the individual, his family, and the community. Work relief,

whatever its defects, supplies some of the accoutrements
of working and at least challenges the decay of men.

The unemployed man, traumatized by the loss of his job,
and, in a lesser way, constantly rejected and put on by
"authority" (refusals of requests for clothes, the unending
intrusion on his privacy by the investigators, the atmosphere
of suspicion about irregular earnings, etc.) comes to still
further defensive anxieties. He is increasingly afraid to
tackle a new job: maybe he has lost his skills, he has no
decent clothes and looks so shabby that he is certain he will
be turned away on that account, he needs a haircut and
can't afford it; he has been turned away so often before he
even had a chance to ask; what will be the attitude of his
fellow workmen, and worst of all, perhaps he will again be
fired. All these fears mount with the passing of time: un-
challenged they threaten complete withdrawal to the group
of permanently unemployed. Whatever it lacks, work relief
at least, offers some of that challenge.

A most important aspect of our problem, one that presses
on the younger unemployed man and his wife is the question whether or not they should have a family. Religious
practices and economics for the moment aside, the limitation on the size of the family poses restrictions, which are
certainly not emotionally healthy for the individual.

A number of families did have children after they had
come on relief: 14 Catholic, 5 Protestant, and 1 Jewish
family. It must be remembered that in addition to their
religious objections to birth control, the Catholics were a
younger group. All the Protestant and the one Jewish family
had children only after a return to private employment had
raised expectations of their renewed independence; hopes
which proved premature.

An aspect of this question of interest to us as psychiatrists is the authorities' refusal to contemplate it at all officially. No allowance is made in the budget for contraceptives, leading in most instances to the use of abstinence or withdrawal as contraceptive methods. Relatively few women knew how to get help from contraceptive clinics, and at least in New York, the investigators of the Department of Welfare were expected to avoid suggesting the use of such resources. Condoms represented a luxury beyond the reach of the unemployed.

A further handicap to normal sexual functioning is imposed by the housing conditions. In 30 of the 60 Home Relief cases serious overcrowding existed, allowing the adults little if any privacy. This, in turn, raised the problem of the exposure of growing children to parental intercourse; many of our parents sensed the problem and made every effort to prevent such episodes. The housing situation made this a problem of restraint and no little ingenuity.

There are many more aspects of the problem of the unemployed: we have attempted to suggest but a few.

What, after years of unemployment, was the attitude of these people to the future? Six didn't want to think of it at all, it was too painful; 5 didn't want to talk about it, although they discussed other matters freely; 17 were fairly optimistic about getting back into private employment, 18 were undecided (really afraid to hope), and 25 were pessimistic. For their children, 18 were optimistic, 33 uneasy and worried, 5 pessimistic.

We came to the end of this study impressed that a group from the beginning underprivileged, faced with an acute and extreme crisis, could make so adequate an adjustment, calling on all their human reserve and resources. We felt, as did Anna Freud after watching the bombed-out British: "We have seen plenty of evil in the world, but one can have only respect and admiration for human beings."

9. THE ROLE OF WORK

WE LIVE in a work-conscious and work-oriented world; indeed, the stereotype of the hustling, ever busy, go-getting American is now an accepted picture of our culture. The American dream is one of social and economic advancement through one's own efforts and our youth is still taught that hard work can accomplish miracles and earnest effort destroy the barriers of class and caste distinction. One of our highest American values is that of success, especially when achieved through the sweat of one's own efforts.

When we consider the central importance that work occupies in the life of the individual and of the group, it is remarkable how little attention psychiatry and psychoanalysis have given to the subject. Whatever attention has been afforded the problem of work has largely dealt with clinical questions such as the neurotic inhibitions of work, compulsive work patterns, and the like; the major theoretical contributions number less than a dozen. This, incidentally, is in sharp contrast to the immense literature on the subject which has been developed by sociology and general psychology. As in other areas of our patients' life stories, the therapist's attention is understandably directed primarily to the nature of the conflict situation, and the role of work in the patient's life is considered only as conflicts interfere with his capacity to perform his work or to derive the usual satisfactions from it. Thus we can say that the practical limitations of the therapeutic situation have largely defined the limits of psychoanalytical concern with the problem of work.

During the past 15 years it has been my privilege to be associated with a group of social scientists concerned with the general problem of work. As a result of this opportunity, I have come to appreciate the validity of considering this entire question in the framework of the reality situation; of relating the dynamic psychological insights gained from the study of the individual to the concept of a person working in a social group and influenced by group values, standards, and goals. With such a concept of the work problem it would, of course, be impossible to encompass the entire subject in a single paper. Hence, I have chosen only two aspects of it: one, the question of occupational choice, which, in a sense, is the point of departure for one's work life; and two, what I should like to call the ego preservative function of work. The latter should interest us especially as therapists since it has much to do with work adjustment and with the evaluation of the individual in his work-a-day world. The following comments are based largely on the results of our joint research, much of which has been published in various places but has not been presented from the point of view I should like to emphasize.

Psychoanalytical contributions to the understanding of the process of occupational choice have never been gathered into a systematic statement but consist largely of incidental observations and comments of varying degrees of explicitness. In general, they fall into three types of explanation.

In the first place, there are the attempts to establish a link

between the present occupation and some significant infantile conflict or impulse, such as that of the builder of
bridges and dams who had difficulties as a child in establishing control over micturition [1] or the surgeon who used to
cut off the tails of neighborhood dogs.[2]

Let us look for a moment at Deutsch's illustration of the
surgeon. She remarks, "One early summer morning many
years ago, the inhabitants of a small German university
town—I think it was Würzburg—made the horrifying discovery that all the dogs which had been running loose during the night in a certain part of the city had lost their tails.
They learned that the medical students had attended a
drinking bout that night and that when they left the party
one young man had had the highly humorous inspiration
to cut off the tails of the dogs. Later he became one of the
most famous surgeons in the world."

While granting the significance of the relationship between the unconscious forces responsible for his earlier
alcoholic exploits and his subsequent career as a surgeon,
a large number of highly important questions remain to be
considered: how and when and why did he choose surgery
from the whole gamut of vocational possibilities which
might equally well have served as gratification for this particular instinctual need (butcher, professional soldier, etc.);
what was the role played by his capacities, aptitudes, skills
and by opportunities for obtaining the necessary education
and training, and could he possibly have gone on to become "one of the most famous surgeons in the world" without these qualities and opportunities, no matter how intense the demand to satisfy an unconscious instinctual
need? The answers to these questions bring the problem
of occupational choice well within the range of considerations of ego functions.

The second type of traditional explanation of why people choose certain occupations rests on the readily ascer-

tainable fact that certain vocations offer opportunities for
the satisfaction of particular needs which exist more or less
consciously in an unmodified form and which may be
more pronounced in some individuals than in others. In
this category would fall the actor whose profession can
satisfy his narcissistic or exhibitionistic needs; the teacher
in a boy's school who has opportunities for homosexual
contacts; the traveling salesman who can indulge in promiscuity with an added safety factor, etc. Similarly, it has
been postulated that the choice of certain occupations rests
primarily on the opportunity such work offers for the expression of other heightened unconscious needs, as scopto-
philic needs in lavatory attendants, destructive sadistic needs
in lumberjacks, etc., or of overwhelming neurotic needs,
as the choice of outdoor work by claustrophobics, etc. I
realize that some of these illustrations bring us to the periphery of the pathological. Any distinction between the
relatively normal and seemingly pathological choices involves largely quantitative factors and does not reflect any
basic difference in the choice process.

Finally, there is a third set of hypotheses, stated or implied, which see in a person's chosen work an essential component in the defensive structure of the personality, usually
in the form of a reaction formation against some heightened
instinctual impulse or unresolved conflict. The social worker's helping role is commonly offered as an example of
the need to insure control of strong original aggression;
Deutsch's dog-tail cutting surgeon would be another.

I look on such explanations as, at best, only partial and
lacking to the extent they fail to take into consideration the
ego factors which play so important a role in the choice of
an occupation. I cannot here describe in any detail our
concept of the choice process but would like to review
briefly some of its salient points. You will find that they
differ with the traditional psychoanalytical explanations

mentioned earlier, explanations which depend almost solely on the role of partial instinctual gratifications. These comments are based on the data gathered in a study of the process of occupational choice, the basic results of which have already been published.[3]

Already in the young child of two or three one sees the important role of ego satisfactions in such activities as the mastery of simple tasks—standing, walking, regularity of toilet practices, the earliest uses of language, etc.; such accomplishments contain within themselves early prototypes of basic patterns involved in the process of occupational choice. Similarly there are the important tasks assigned to young children; emptying the ash trays or helping set the table, etc. In addition to the opportunity of sharing a task with a loved person and achieving praise through accomplishment, there is the important and highly relevant factor of ego satisfaction in the mastery of the assigned task itself. Erikson [4] tells an unusually felicitous story to illustrate the point that even in the young child the "ego identity gains real strength only from whole-hearted and consistent recognition of real accomplishment. Dr. Ruth Underhill tells me of sitting with a group of Papago elders in Arizona when the man of the house turned to his little three-year-old granddaughter and asked her to close the door. The door was heavy and hard to shut. The child tried but it did not move. Several times the grandfather repeated, 'Yes, close the door.' No one jumped to the child's assistance. No one took the responsibility away from her. On the other hand there was no impatience, for after all the child was small. They sat gravely waiting until the child succeeded and her grandfather gravely thanked her. It was assumed that the task would not be asked of her unless she could perform it and having been asked, the responsibility was hers alone just as if she were a grown woman."

The child on the threshold of puberty first becomes aware of the fact that the task of choosing his future work rests with him and that he must sooner or later accept responsibility for the choice. Before this the child usually believes that he will do and be whatever his father, mother, teacher, or some other idealized person suggests; his main motivation at this time is the need to strengthen his ego by a close identification with a strong, loved object and the hope that in compliance he can gain love and approval and avoid the weighty responsibility of independent decision. Gradually it begins to dawn on him that he may not like any of the things suggested; that he may not be interested in them. Only then does he begin to look for and ultimately find a firm basis for his formal choice, namely in his *own* interests.

With increasing maturity reality factors enter the picture in a second step which requires the use of the ego's reality testing functions to clarify the choice of alternatives. Value considerations also begin to exert their influence, thereby complicating the process still further. Considerable anxiety may be aroused in the youngster, especially during adolescence, while he tries to clarify his choice.

In his efforts to accomplish this goal, the youngster's awareness and estimate of his interests occupy a central place. My colleagues and I look on interests as powerful forces in the personality which undoubtedly are derived from deeper instinctual sources and which carry with them the hallmarks of instincts in that they become powerful motives in their own right—autonomous, if you wish— and the satisfaction of which affords the individual a considerable premium of pleasure. We believe them to be genuine examples of sublimation and closely allied to other ego functions, notably the intellectual ones. They are developed on the basis of identification with grownups and peers and constitute, we believe, a fusion of libidinal and aggressive components. It should also be emphasized that interests are closely tied to capacities; it is almost impossible to maintain over any extended period of time an interest for which one lacks capacity. However, self-evaluation with regard to capacities comes into play quite late, in our observation roughly around fourteen or fifteen. Apparently the heightened narcissism during puberty prevents the adolescent from gaining a sufficient degree of distance from himself before then, and the ego is not yet equal to the often quite painful task of self-examination. It is clear that self-evaluation is subject to interference not only from narcissism, but also from disturbances in the regulation of self-esteem, and many other factors which make for insecurity and anxiety about one's self. It should be emphasized, of course, that many adults fail to achieve a reasonably accurate self-evaluation, especially where talent is concerned.

A third step in the development of the occupational choice process is reached around sixteen or seventeen when the youngster considers his future work in the wider framework of his life plan, his goals and values. Shortly thereafter he becomes aware of an increasing need for a more complete range of experience which he hopes to find through increasing reality testing during his early college years, or, in case of those who leave school, by trying out various kinds of work.

To summarize very briefly: we look on the choice of an occupation as a process involving, as in other compromise solutions, the individual's desire to find in work an outlet for instinctual needs which will also meet the demands of his superego and comply with the various ego requirements that are involved. The ego, here as in other processes, has the important defensive aspect, so well summarized by Anna Freud: [5] "The ego is victorious when its defensive measures effect their purpose, i.e., when they enable it to restrict the development of anxiety and pain and so to transform the instincts that, even in difficult circumstances, some measure of gratification is secured, thereby establishing the most harmonious relations possible between the id, the superego and the forces of the outside world." However, beyond such purely defensive needs, a successful occupational choice must lead to work which will provide the wealth of potential ego satisfactions, some of which have been suggested here: mastery of the assigned task, satisfying job (work) social relations; fulfillment of the adult and appropriate sexual roles, gains in prestige and rewards, and others. These ego satisfactions are basic, consequential, and necessary to an adequate work adjustment.

This brings us to the second problem area I have chosen for discussion, a consideration of what I have called the ego-preservative function of work. As therapists, we naturally have a great interest in this aspect of work, bearing directly as it does on our everyday activities.

I have long been interested in noting how often experience seems to bear out my earlier clinical impression that many people who are disturbed emotionally and mentally continue to work even though seriously ill and that they hold on to their work longer than to many other important tasks of life. And, further, that the disturbance will often remain unnoticed on the job long after family and friends have noticed serious disintegration in the patient's personal and social relationships. (I recognize, of course, that the opposite can and does occur and that in specific instances an individual will give up his work as the first external evidence of an illness.) To check on this impression, I went over the records of my private cases for two separate years, 1943 and 1952. Choosing men between the ages of twenty and fifty-five, I had usable records on some fifty-five patients. Of these, five were actually psychotic; the remainder included the usual run of neurotic, psychopathic, and so-called borderline states. Of the fifty, only four were unable to work on their jobs or were doing badly; fourteen were not aware of any interference whatsoever in their work habits, their performance, or level of satisfaction. Two of the four with work interference had sought help on that account. These are merely approximate figures and no degree of statistical validity is intended.

Naturally people who seek private help represent a rather biased sample as to economic and social status, the kind of work they do, and, in part, their level of accomplishment and innate capacities. To correct this bias somewhat a member of the staff took two samples, of fifty cases each, from two outpatient clinics in New York City. As we expected, the proportion of people who were totally incapacitated in regard to their ability to work was considerably higher. However, the proportion was still remarkably small —less than twenty per cent—and a considerable number of the most disturbed patients in this group were working. We cannot, of course, consider these results conclusive, in view of the selective factors which operate for admission to an outpatient clinic.

Granting the validity of my clinical impression, what answers are available to explain it? Two possibilities suggest themselves on the basis of general analytic considerations, and, indeed, they have already been mentioned by Hart.[6] One is that work affords an opportunity for the discharge and binding of a multitude of instinctual tendencies, narcissistic, partial instinctual, object libidinal, and aggressive. This is true enough, but it seems doubtful that it really answers the question because such an explanation does not consider why disturbances in the economy of libidinal and aggressive drives which are caused by interferences with discharge through normal channels should not equally affect the discharge of these impulses through work activity.

One possible solution to this dilemma may be the hypothesis that work can more easily be isolated from the rest of the personality, but then we would have to explain why this degree of isolation can be greater in the case of work than in other functions.

The second suggestion to be found in analytical literature speaks of work in relation to the system of defense. The compulsive worker is generally used as an example to demonstrate this. In this instance work has the character of a symptom and hence constitutes a form of discharge of instinctual energies which simultaneously meet the demands of the superego. Here, too, the fact is beyond doubt, but the explanation is incomplete so long as it does not state why instinctual satisfaction expressed in terms of work is capable of meeting these superego demands when other forms of satisfaction are interdicted. In the case of compulsive work, analytical theory can readily supply a model for the missing link in the explanation. In terms of the instinctual impulses, be they libidinal or aggressive, their utilization in work means that they no longer pursue their original aim, i.e., that they have been neutralized. In terms of the ego, they have become part of it. They have been attached to specific ego functions which act as carriers of these sublimated instinctual energies, or, we may say, they have been appropriated by the ego for its own use. The resistive character of work activities can then be understood on the basis of this transformation of id impulses into ego energies, allowing of course for the possibility, and likelihood, that the many activities and contacts with people in the course of working offer opportunities for the discharge of various instinctual impulses in a more direct fashion. Many of these present themselves incidentally and constitute what may be designated as concomitant work satisfactions. These sublimated instinctual energies enter into the formation of play and work activities alike and make them actually part of the very structure of the ego. There are other aspects of work which show how closely allied work activity is to essential ego functions. Foremost among them is the fact that work is directed toward reality; it aims at changing it. Freud [7] said, "Laying stress upon the importance of work has a greater effect on binding the individual more closely to reality than any other technique of living." He also gives due weight to the social factor in work when he points out that: "In his work he (the individual) is at least securely attached to a part of reality, the human community." But beyond pointing out that this factor is intimately connected with work satisfactions, I shall not be able to elaborate on this concept at this time.

In addition, work occupies a central position in the formation of the structure of the ego, because it is one of the most important visible manifestations of adulthood; [8] in other words, it is a major vehicle of identification with the role of the adult. Actually, this goes beyond simple ego functions inasmuch as it includes the relationship of work to the ego-ideal. Hence, losing the ability to work threatens the ego, not only in terms of its contact with reality, and in the loosening of its social bonds, but, more basically, in regard to its relationship to the ego-ideal as well.

As a matter of fact, most of our work attitudes are under the command of the superego. On the other hand, such aspects of our work-a-day life as the routinized character of many of our work activities, attendance, regularity, meeting standards of performance, and even the avoidance of such indulgences as, for example, drinking, are demands which are made on us not only by the superego but also by the outside world. Therefore, it can be said that meeting

these demands from the outside acts as a support to the
ego when the superego is too weak to enforce compliance;
in much the same way as parental demands and supervision
strengthen the as yet weak superego of the child who is
tempted by the pleasures of play when he should be doing
his homework.

Taken in their totality, the orientation to reality, the
maintenance of social bonds, the identification with the
adult role, and meeting specific superego demands sup-
ported by demands from the outside—these factors constitute an important part of the function of the ego. From
which it can be concluded that the person who is threatened
by the destructive forces emerging from the unconscious
would want to hold on to work because abandoning it
means abandoning ego control and surrender to these forces.
Thus, keeping the work function intact as long as possible
is a major bulwark against the tendencies toward regres-
sion. An ancient sage, asked to explain why Adam had
died, said, "He died because he no longer worked." By
this he meant that living entirely for one's self (we would
say: entirely by the pleasure principle) is not enough; one
must live for others and in the actual world (by the reality
principle) as well. If you build a house, till a field, teach
the young, your work is reality oriented and extends beyond mere pleasure and, hence, sustains life. To have work
to do is to be needed and to be needed is essential for life.
Just in passing, I should like to point out that this ancient
concept clearly corroborates our modern doubts about the
practice of compulsory retirement.

The extent and the value of the support which is derived
from the external demands of the usual work setting can
be seen clearly when one considers situations where they
are absent. Take, for example, people who work alone and
independently (scientists, artists, and others); who have to

rely entirely on their own self-discipline because they have
no work place to go to, no regular office hours, no dead-
lines to meet, no standards of performance to uphold save
their own. This is especially true if, in addition, their livelihood does not directly depend on their work. It is well-
known that such people find it harder to maintain work
discipline and become more easily victims of work disturbances.

   The isolated worker usually has none of these external
supports to fall back on and the creative person has, in
addition, a greater dependence on processes which are closer
to the unconscious than the average worker. He is more
dependent in his work on inspiration, it is closer to phantasy
than reality and its relationship to the "human community"
is both more indirect and more tenuous; consisting at times
of not much more than the vague hope of fame or recognition in some indeterminate future, perhaps not even within
his lifetime. What helps him to overcome these obstacles
are the very forces which make him a creative person: (1)
he is driven to work by these very forces of the unconscious
which give rise to his inspiration (which corresponds to
the discharge factor mentioned earlier); (2) the objectification of these impulses in the form of creative work, be it
artistic or scientific, falls into the category of more highly
valued products as compared to the usual products of work,
at least in terms of his own value scheme; (3) the intensity
of work satisfaction in the act of creation is undoubtedly
greater and involves the totality of his being in a more profound sense than everyday kinds of work, even when the
act of creation itself is a painful one; and, finally, (4) in
creative work, narcissism plays a greater role than in other
kinds of work. The heightened narcissism is recognizable
in the greater reliance on phantasy and in the looser connection with physical and social reality; it is not only a

more powerful motive and a more intense gratification if
and when recognition is accorded him; it is also invested
to a greater degree with his own standards of performance.
Let us now turn to a brief discussion of people who have
no work, in light of our hypothesis about the ego-preservative function of work. The observations on which these
remarks are based have been published in an earlier book
on the unemployed.[9] To the man who is unemployed, the
loss of work is obviously a threat to survival, mitigated somewhat by social measures devised for his protection; it is
also a severe threat to the integration of his personality.

Lacking all the instinctual satisfactions that are gained in
work, and deprived of the ego supports and satisfactions
of the work situation both in their individual and social
aspects, the unemployed person is threatened with a virtual
emasculation in any effective functional sense. Nor is he
capable of arriving at that degree of internal equilibrium
which is afforded the disturbed person through the formation of his symptoms. In fact, my colleagues and I found
that, contrary to what might have been expected, there
was no tendency among the unemployed to resort to illness; nor was there any increase in such regressive phenomena as promiscuity, masturbation, criminality, or alcoholism. The only change in the sexual behaviour of these
men that we could detect was a somewhat more frequent
indulgence in intercourse, expressing a greater need for
maintaining masculine prerogatives.

As we came to know the individuals who constituted our
sample in the study of what unemployment does to people,
we found that psychological reactions which in other circumstances would have had pathological significance turned
out, in this instance, to be temporary protective devices.
They would while away their time at such activities as
making toys for their children out of kitchenware. But this

was not idle play. By making these toys they remained the
father, the provider. And even the switch in social-sexual
roles to which some of the men turned appeared to be only
an attempt to stabilize a disturbed internal equilibrium. In
assuming the feminine role by doing housework, etc., they
protected themselves against having no role to play. While
they could not entirely escape the threat of mobilizing
castration anxiety by this reversal of role, they were com-
pensated for it by maintaining their self-esteem in terms
of assuming some responsibilities of the adult, rather than
permitting themselves to fall into the role of total dependency. Also the almost Quixotic search for work which was
simply not to be found during the 1930s can be understood
in the light of these considerations. As long as a man tried
to find work he did what he could to safeguard his adult
masculine role, to behave like a man in our society. It is
interesting and of the greatest importance to note that these
self-protective devices of the unemployed men turned out
to be entirely reversible, that is, when they finally did find
work all of these modifications of their personality fell
away and they soon re-established their original personality
structures.

   If we ask ourselves how the unemployed could withstand
the pressures arising from their predicament, we must consider two factors in addition to the individual devices of
self-protection just mentioned. One is the strengthening of
the bond of social solidarity through the material support
given them by society, which in some measure helped them
to feel that they were not considered worthless, even though
they did not earn the money. The other was their awareness that theirs was not an individual fate nor one for which
they needed to feel guilty but that they were victims of
a social calamity, over which they had no control.

   What I have reported are some thoughts about two

aspects of the complex phenomenon known as work. As therapists, we naturally must have great interest in a part of life which for men, and increasingly for many women, constitutes a primary and inescapable daily demand. Traditionally, we try to understand adjustment *from within*, so to speak; that is, in terms of the inner dynamic forces responsible for adjustment and maladjustment to situations outside the individual. Work adjustment, in a sense, is a "public" matter, in contrast to, let us say, sexual adjustment, and to study it requires a public laboratory different from the hospital or the psychiatrist's office. It is to be hoped that such studies as these will take the concern about work adjustment out of its narrow clinical boundaries and seek understandings which in turn may be used effectively in therapeutic situations. To take a single instance: the adjustment of the worker to his job must reflect such supportive elements as job security, opportunities for socializing, as well as inner tensions which he may project on to the job situation from other aspects of life. A fuller understanding of the nature and consequence of the interplay between the external forces, especially the ego supportive ones, and the inner dynamics may well be put to work in helping people to adjust, especially where deeper understanding may not be available to the individual. Such advances will require an ever broadening concept of psychiatry as a social science.

IO. WORK AND ITS SATISFACTIONS

MY EARLY clinical experiences with work problems were quite unexceptional and provided no special stimulus to my interest in this subject. I saw the occasional but hardly rare patient who complained of some vague feeling of dissatisfaction with his job, of a special work inhibition or of compulsive work habits or special needs in working conditions. Like most of my colleagues I approached these problems entirely from the point of view of the individual, viewing them, not without justification, as expressions of neurotic conflicts in the patients' work life, quite analogous to problems in sexual behavior, marital adjustment, somatic functioning, etc.

Nor had theory greatly catalyzed my interest in work. The explicit writings in the psychoanalytic literature on work were, as indeed they remain, meager, just as Freud's references to work are casual and are made largely in passing while discussing other and presumably more consequential matters. In this connection it is interesting to note how many of Freud's comments on work are made in footnotes.

Gradually, my clinical experience challenged certain of these accepted notions, and increasingly I became aware of dimensions in the problem of work that seemed to demand further investigation and explanation. Thus, quite early I found it difficult to accept the notion of man's natural aversion to work as I found repeated evidence of a driving need to work, independent of economic need or the quest for prestige and status or other such easily discernible motivations.

My attention was first vividly drawn to this dimension of the work problem when the father of a young patient of mine consulted me about his son. He was a youthful, middle-aged man, not yet fifty, who had nominally retired some years previously to attend to the family's inherited wealth and to "loaf." As I got to know him better I was struck by the work aspects of his life: his almost endless round of board meetings, his intense "volunteer" activities on behalf of his prep school. Even in his "loafing" he devoted meticulous attention to detail in such matters as outfitting and completing arrangements for his big-game hunting or deep-sea fishing expeditions, and exercised the greatest care in choosing the personnel for these trips. I was especially impressed when he returned from one of these safaris quite exhausted, if exhilarated by the "bag," to say to me, by way of a joke, that if he continued to be so tired he thought he would have to retire "back to work."

My practice provided other illustrations of attitudes toward work which aroused my interest: the special work circumstances and problems of creative and scientific workers; the often difficult to understand sources of pleasure and satisfaction in bizarre and, to the observer, unrewarding work situations; the fact that some people were able to work quite adequately, to judge by performance, even in the presence of severe, debilitating emotional illness whereas, in others, the limitation in capacity to work was almost the first evidence of such illness.

At any rate, when in 1939 it was my privilege to join

a team of social scientists then, as now, under the direction of Dr. Eli Ginzberg, in a study of the unemployed, I was eager to have an opportunity to investigate some of the less directly clinical aspects of the work problem.[1] This began a long and, I believe, fruitful cooperative effort to study various aspects of these and related questions, which is still in progress, though it has broadened out into many bypaths on the way. It was our belief that since in medicine one learned much about the normal from a study of the pathological, a study of the "sickest" element of the working community, those excluded from it entirely and through circumstances over which they exercised no control whatsoever, would provide insights into the complicated problems connected with work, especially the sources of satisfaction in work.

The details of this study have been published,[2] but it was interesting to review them at this extraordinarily different period in our history, especially in the light of more recent developments in our knowledge of the psychological aspects of work. Although all of us who participated in this study had known these families in a curiously intimate way, they now seemed quite unreal, so thoroughly have we succeeded in repressing the painful details of the depression years. The specter of the apple vendor on our street corners seems as distant as a character in a Hogarth drawing. It is difficult to re-create the social unrest and individual plight of those years, and a whole generation has grown up for whom such symbols as WPA are only historical fragments.

Here was a heterogeneous group of men cut off from their usual course of income and their customary way of life by a social crisis which precipitated them and their families into a frightening dependence on governmental and charitable aid. Every aspect of their lives was inevitably altered, and although no one faced the ultimate disaster of starvation, they were all—men, women and children—involved in a life experience of deprivation and social isolation of the greatest depth and consequence. Studying these unemployed men, we realized increasingly that the meaning of a man's work could be understood only in the broader context of his whole life, and that work satisfactions represented something more than the factors commonly emphasized at that time, such as pleasures attached to body function, the expression of repressed unconscious instinctual needs or partial instinct gratifications, important as these may be to a given individual. In fact, our experience led us to appreciate Freud's [3] estimate of the importance of work as attaching the worker securely to a part of reality, "the human community."

Many elements go into work thus considered. In the first place, work defines one's place in the society, emphasizes one's feelings of usefulness and belonging, and is a constantly renewed sign that one is not left out of the scheme of things. The common routine in which workers are involved is of itself an important ego-strengthening device. It provides a structure and gives direction to their waking hours.[4]

It is now commonly stated that most workers are quite dissatisfied with their work, that the worker lives in an "alienated" world, and that he simply resigns himself to his job because there is no escape. I shall come back to a consideration of this contention. For the unemployed man any such emphasis on lack of satisfaction in a job—any job—would have seemed an unbelievable abstraction, and if a man occasionally verbalized discontent with his last job, it was plainly to try to cushion the painful impact of his joblessness, and to minimize the vastness of his feeling of loss and deprivation.

Another important trauma suffered by the unemployed

man was the threat to his status in the role of the father, authority figure in the household. Work is a vital and basic instrument whereby one achieves and maintains one's role and status in the family group; security and pleasure in this role are an indirect but basic part of a man's work "satisfaction." The importance of this matter of status and family role takes on a new perspective in light of the increasing number of women who work and of their changing position in the family structure. Unfortunately, I cannot discuss this here because of space limitations.

It was not surprising to find that such a castrating blow as severance from one's job should often result in one of two types of behavior: (1) the effort to assert feelings of genital adequacy and hence to make excessive sexual demands, if one used the man's previous attitudes as the norm; or (2) a retreat into resigned, feminine attitudes and the shift of the parental, decision-making authority to the woman. The woman's attitudes toward sexual intercourse also reflected the loss of the man's role as the father-authority figure in the household. Many of them who had tolerated their husbands' sexual advances now withdrew entirely: "When my husband was working and supporting me and the family it was right for him to have sexual relations and I tolerated it. Now I don't have to any longer." For many of these men, the impact of this catastrophe was too overwhelming and they retreated into a passive dependent attitude. Certain of these efforts were clearly designed to reduce conscious feelings of unworthiness and self-denigration and to expiate for the feelings of guilt created by the man's awareness of his incapacity to fulfill his masculine role. One is not surprised, in this connection, to note how little comfort was afforded by the conscious appreciation of the man's blamelessness and how the current reality situation was used to channelize other unconscious sources of guilt.

It is of some clinical interest to note that little somatic illness was present in the sample of unemployed men we studied. This was surely a tension- and anxiety-producing crisis, with great and inescapable feelings of frustration, theoretically calculated to result in such illnesses as hypertension, ulcer formation, etc. Except for the rare instance of alcoholism, whose beginnings were clearly present long before the men became unemployed, there were only rare instances of illness in which one might discern psychogenic elements.

As I stated, it is a far cry from these considerations of the unemployed man of the depression years to the opinions now current, especially in the writings of contemporary industrial psychologists and sociologists, that work is lacking in satisfaction because of the alienated work world; in fact one might infer that work is a barren "curse," demoralizing and destructive in its influences on the workers. This notion that work represents a "curse" [5] for most people is one which I cannot easily accept and which, as I hope to demonstrate, is hardly tenable on either theoretical or practical grounds.

In the first place, any such idea must reflect some idealized concept of work which is then used as a baseline for comparison. In the orthodox Christian concept, work is a sacred duty to God and thus becomes a thing apart, rewarded for its holiness and hence above such concerns as wages, etc. One does see such attitudes toward work in certain special social groups. A striking illustration of this is in the Kibbutzim society in Israel, where *hakkara* (literally "consciousness") "requires" a special dedication to work. Especially in those settlements where no private property, money, rewards, etc., exist, where there is no supervision of any worker by a superior nor anyone to check on him, no clock to punch and no hours arbitrarily prescribed, motivation for work rests entirely in the individual's *hakkara*, his awareness and acceptance of his role as worker in a community. "His job . . . becomes more than a job and more than a way of making a living. It becomes a *sacred task*, a calling, in the religious sense of that term, dedicated not to the greater glory of God but to the welfare of the group." [6]

To expect any such devotion to work or any such order of satisfaction from work by an ordinary worker smacks of a high degree of romantic unrealism. And yet it seems that the social scientists, now that they have begun to ask workers how they feel about their jobs, tend to plot their findings against some such unreal standard. One might ask what the peasants in earlier times, or the hand-loom workers of a later period, let alone the slaves, would have answered to the questionnaires currently in use and how the answers of present-day workers would measure up against them.

It was, incidentally, a tacit acceptance of the notion that workers considered their work a curse and worked for money alone that led to many of the confusions encountered earlier concerning the unemployed, since it was widely assumed that if their dollar security could be maintained they would prefer not to work. But such was surely not the case among many of the unemployed whom we studied. Here were men who continued to put forth much physical and even more emotional effort to search for a job, for any kind of work, even in the face of overwhelming evidence that work was not to be found. It could be said, too simply and glibly, that they were compulsive and driven by some inner necessity in this quest for work. A small widening of our concept of "necessity" would, in a sense, make this applicable to all of us; such are the superego requirements for work in our world. But this is a far cry from equating work with a curse.

In a previous work,[7] we have considered the complex

problem of work satisfaction from a rather different but closely related point of view. This study undertook to evaluate and describe the process whereby one chooses one's life work and the emotional and other commitments such a choice demands of an individual. Such investments, especially the emotional ones, reflect an individual's values, goals and life expectations, and play a tremendous role in future work satisfactions. Stated briefly, we distinguished three major components: returns, including earnings, intrinsic satisfactions, and concomitant satisfactions.[8]

Every person is interested, at least to some degree, in monetary returns. He must earn enough to maintain himself, and usually a family, even if he is willing to accept a low standard of living. With respect to intrinsic satisfactions, the variation among people may be considerably greater, although at present we know little about this. Probably many people are willing to engage in any work that is not actually frustrating; they do not seek intrinsic satisfaction. If a job is tolerable, their primary concern is with the salary or wages and the general conditions under which they work. With respect to the conditions of work, most people can probably adjust to a rather wide range. On the other hand, for many, environment is important and may lead to either satisfaction or frustration. They compromise by accepting lower returns in order to work in a satisfactory environment. Even exceptional returns would not induce some of them to work under unacceptable conditions.

Any such conceptualization of the problem obviously allows for great individual and cultural variations.

My thoughts on work satisfactions were again stimulated when I was recently asked to discuss a paper which was not given but which was to have the title: "Work and the Escape from Self." In the absence of a script I decided to speculate on what the author could mean by this title, and, drawing on our work on the unemployed, on occupational choice, and on a larger and as yet unpublished monograph on the meaning of work, I entertained these notions. (I naturally have no idea if they in any way resemble the author's unread ones.)

"Self" would in the first instance place the emphasis on ego factors, and the title hence implies that work has become ego-alien or ego-frustrating. It is not plain to me why that should be more true now than previously, if indeed it is true at all. The binding quality of work certainly is undiminished and its value as the most important link to reality is unchanged. Freud [9] assigned to the ego "the task of bringing the influence of the external world to bear upon the id and its tendencies and endeavors to substitute the reality principle for the pleasure principle which reigns supreme in the id." Work is obviously one of the main devices whereby the healthy ego accomplishes this result. As Erikson [10] has pointed out, before the child can become a biological parent,

. . . he must begin to be a worker and potential provider. With the oncoming latency period, the normally advanced child forgets, or rather sublimates, the necessity to "make" people by direct attack or to become papa and mama in a hurry: he now learns to win recognition by producing things. He has mastered the ambulatory field and the organ modes. He has experienced a sense of finality regarding the fact that there is no workable future within the womb of his family, and thus becomes ready to apply himself to given skills and tasks, which go far beyond the mere playful expression of his organ modes or the pleasure in the function of his limbs. He develops industry—i.e., he adjusts himself to the inorganic laws of the tool world. He can become an eager and absorbed unit of a productive situation. To bring a productive situation to completion is an aim which gradually supersedes the whims and wishes of his autonomous organism. His ego boundaries include his tools and skills: the work principle (Ives Hendrick) teaches him the pleasure of work completion by steady attention and persevering diligence.

It is exactly in the area of work that "the ego's tendency to turn passivity into activity thus acquires a new field of manifestation, in many ways superior to the mere turning of passive into active in infantile fantasy and play; for now the inner need for activity, practice and work completion is ready to meet the corresponding demands and opportunities in social reality." [11]

The concepts of denial of self, of alienation in work, seemingly represent the notion of a withdrawal of cathexis from work. Such a denial must hypothecate either a high order of frustration and lack of satisfaction in work or, perhaps, the presence of more available and more satisfying channels for libidinal gratification.

Much is made of the fact that modern work conditions (and this applies essentially to factory machine-belt type of work) do not make it possible for a worker to participate in the whole of a given work operation or to bring to completion an entire task of production, but rather to participate only in a fraction of the process.

There were instances during the war—but so far as I can learn even these were rare—where workers were engaged in making some part or gadget whose ultimate use could not be revealed to them for security reasons. I doubt if in other instances the fact that a worker does only a small part of a larger operation can really be a source of frustration and tension to him, or that it will deny him the narcissistic satisfaction of a well-done "piece of work." He knows perfectly well the purpose of his part of the operation, and if he is at all identified in a positive way with his company and their product that feeling must surely include his share of the operation. A much more important source of frustration and tension on a job might well occur if a man were prevented from using his skills, especially those in whose acquisition he has made a great emotional investment through sacrifices in the training period, etc. Such a lack of opportunity could well be ego denying and, in the extreme, even intolerable.

Such realities as the condition of the physical plant, reasonable pay, etc., are accepted as important; but greater stress is laid on such conditions as fragmentation of work, the failure of management to include the worker in "responsible," i.e., decision-making roles, and on supervision that fails to take into account the worker's need for prestige and status. This sort of concern is reflected in the construction of "morale" scales in which such factors as "I think this company treats its employees better than any other company"; "The company is sincere in wanting to know what its employees think about it"; and "In the long run the company will 'put it over' on you" are variously scored to reach a level of "morale." Such scales and similar techniques seem incredibly naïve to a psychoanalyst, conscious of the complexities of motivation and satisfaction. In psychological terms they obviously are concerned with certain lacks of narcissistic and ego satisfactions. I do not know the basis for the concept that a worker seeks his narcissistic gratifications solely or even primarily in his job. In fact, there is substantial evidence that for most industrial workers, work and the work setting are not central life interests.[12] There may very well be a considerable loss of ego gratification to the modern worker who does not find the same order of satisfaction in the shared interests, the comradeship with fellow workers, etc., that were characteristic of former generations. How great this loss actually is remains to be determined.

In the first place, it is assumed that for some undefined

reason work must be creative, challenging or highly rewarding in emotional terms to make it meaningful. Few men
are ever creative; ordinary work never has been creative
and there is no reason to expect it to be different today. The
same kind of comment might be made about the concept
that because men are not given responsibility on their jobs
they are, therefore, frustrated. On the contrary, we know
that in general people shun responsibility, for with it go
risks, including the risk of failure.

I know of no evidence for such a statement as this: "The
preference for a job which offers greater 'security,' spurious
as it may be, is due to neurotic insecurity. . . ." Security is
rated highly among all workers, and this seems to me understandable and the expression of a prevailing human need.
Perhaps in our world only artists and migrant workers are
exempt from this need for security.

Actually, the areas of satisfaction available to workers are
wider now than ever. We have come from an average work
week of 70 to 80 hours to one of 35 to 40 and, on the average,
the worker has much more free income to spend. There
are many important areas of satisfaction made possible by
this shift. Principally, I would point out a really new opportunity for working fathers to participate in family living
and to share the joys and satisfactions attached to such
active participation. I need hardly emphasize the widespread importance of this. Secondly, there is the opportunity for new and varied use of leisure time. I do not share
at all the horror with which such aspects of leisure activity
as looking at TV are viewed. For example: one reads,
"Choices among movies or juke boxes are pseudo-choices
because in either case they represent personality-alien en-
tertainment. They are fixed activities and therefore deaden-
ing; they can only be taken or left, call for no participation,
and cannot be geared to the individual's need or formed by

his total personality." Or, again, "A life may be full of activity and contain a variety of experiences, but it will still seem empty if activities and experiences do not bear the personal flavor of individual choice, taste, appreciation." [13] So long as *free choice* exists I am not alarmed, and would suggest that the improvement of taste had better not be confused with the question of freedom. Sunday mornings in spring and summer I watch fathers of all economic and social groups join their children in the park to play baseball with varying degrees of skill. It happens I share their enthusiasm for baseball and hence value this as an activity. I might not share their appreciation of "I Love Lucy," but I would not be concerned with the freedom of their souls or the deleterious impact on their mental health because they do.

If indeed modern work is, in general, lacking in opportunities for id satisfactions, and if narcissistic gratifications are harder to achieve, it would be understandable that, *given time and money*, the worker looks to the community and his leisure time activities for a good share of the gratification he seeks.

Work offers, now as always, for those who are relatively unhampered by severe emotional problems, a full range of ego, superego, and id satisfactions, varying of course with job and individual. I see no justification for the despair expressed by Chisholm: [14] "Our children should be prepared to bring their children up so they won't have to work as a neurotic necessity. The necessity to work is a neurotic symptom. It is a crutch. It is an attempt to make oneself feel valuable even though there is no particular need for one's working." And to have this heralded as "the true spirit of psychoanalytic theory"! [15]

Work is a basic part of everyone's life. It supplies the means not only to support life, but to afford leisure pursuits which are gratifying and meaningful to the individual. Work is a social activity, and the end products of the worker's efforts have a social value.

What has come to be known as Freud's "shortest saying" says much about this whole problem. He "was once asked what he thought a normal person should be able to do well." He is reported to have said: "Lieben und arbeiten" (to love and to work). Erikson [16] interprets this to mean "a general work-productiveness which would not pre-occupy the individual to the extent that he loses his right or capacity to be a genital and a loving being. Thus," Erikson contends, and I would emphatically agree, "we may ponder, but we cannot improve on the formula which includes the doctor's prescription for human dignity—and for democratic living."

II. THE AMERICAN FAMILY

AS I BEGIN to put down these few comments on American family life I have the uncomfortable feeling that I am about to perpetuate one of the very things of which I am going to complain. It seems certain to me that we suffer from too many self-appointed (and self-anointed) authorities on family life. Almost everyone "gets into the act"—educators, jurists, social scientists, philosophers, economists, psychologists, social workers, psychiatrists. All seem challenged to express themselves authoritatively about what they consider to be wrong with family life, especially in this country. I want to share a quandary with you and speculate a bit about it. How indeed did this preoccupation with the family occur, and how and why is so generally dismal a picture painted of family life in this country?

From the journalistic forays one might begin to wonder if indeed the family were here to stay—but we may be reassured about this. The family is the oldest of social institutions, and though it has altered its size and shape and the method of transacting its affairs as it struggled to meet the new demands that were being made on it, we know it has survived and, indeed—despite the cries of alarm—flourishes. If one were to take the criteria of the market place they would be reassuring: more people marry, over-all at a younger age, and they have more children, than previously. There are, after all, some 42 million families in the country! Of course, this statement requires much refinement to be valid, and we will discuss at least one of the facets that weigh somewhat against a too optimistic use of that statistic.

But I would first divest myself of any cloak of authority on this subject; as a psychoanalyst and the consultant to a flourishing counseling service I naturally hear a great deal about marriage but, especially in private practice, always from the special and highly personalized and idiosyncratic point of view of, so to speak, one or both of the contestants in the match.

In general, the free associative device which psychoanalysis employs more or less precludes the kind of consistent and detailed information a good sociologist, for instance, would consider adequate. Actually, I have long been interested in the special nature and quality of my patients' communications. To begin with they are constrained to bring in what they, at any rate, *think* will please the therapist ("be interesting") and, if often unconsciously, they trim their views to those they hope will be compatible with what they assume is his value system. As Ackerman has emphasized, "A psychiatrist, being primarily a healer, focuses preferentially on the sick parts of human functioning; he accents the negative, pathogenic components of behavior, but sees the residually healthy tendencies less clearly." The understanding of the special communication system—"doctor-therapist"—is a complicated process having many levels of meaning into which we cannot even venture at this time. All I want to do is emphasize my awareness that my special training and experience fit me, if at all, into a casual sort of expertise in family problems.

My experience at the Arthur Lehman Counseling Service, where I am privileged to be a consultant, has in the
last few years offered some measure of corrective to private
practice. Here the problems of family life are bared much
more immediately and inquiry into the sources of tension
made much more directly. I would not, however, feel that
even this experience has made me expert, though it has
indeed sharpened my awareness of some of the problems
that trouble families.

My lack of special training and experience is perhaps
the least of the hazards in my talking about the family.
The American family is such a heterogeneous conglomera-
tion of all classes, castes, ethnic and religious backgrounds,
and regional differences as to make generalizations in this
field especially venturesome. To make one that will apply
with any reasonable accuracy to a New England family
of four or five or more generations in this country, a family
of second generation East European immigrants, a rural
family in the deep South—perhaps still sharecropping for
their livelihood—and the family of a sheep herder in the
Southwest (to pick samples at random and with no special
interest in dramatizing contrasts; other examples could easily
have been found to accomplish this) is a foolhardy and
not particularly fruitful endeavor. And so it must be recognized from the outset that most of these generalizations
are pretty much restricted to urban, middle- and upper
middle-class families now mostly two or more generations
in this country.

The family has a natural history of its own which it
is important to recall. It consists essentially of the relationships between a married couple, husband and wife; between this pair and their children, and among the children
themselves in various sibling relationships. In many cultures this basic core pattern is, of course, vastly different.

Not so long ago in our country grandparents, aunts, uncles, and various cousins would surely have been included and, at the opposite extreme, there are distant cultures which require brother-sister marriages among their royal strains. There is an infinite variety of permitted or expected arrangements in the family in a given culture at a given period. But there are certain generalizations which we may make, if somewhat hesitantly, about the contemporary American family. As I said earlier, increasingly, regardless of class origin, the standards, mores, expectations, and values are those of the middle class.

The American family pattern has been greatly changed by the increase in urbanization, the over-all improvement of our economic and material standards, by the changes in traditional methods of work at home, both in terms of the almost complete disappearance of industrial work done at home by women and by the vast increase in gadgets, improvements in food preparation, etc. Religious worship and practice are no longer the *family* functions they once were, and there has been what Mowrer calls a "loss of family consciousness."

Burgess, a pioneer in this field of family studies, has summarized the changes in family life as follows: a downgrading of the authority of parents; a trend toward egalitarianism in the relations between male and female, with a relative decrease in the authority of the father; parental uncertainty; decline in the importance of grandparents; and the irresponsibility of children. This adds up to a new form of family structure, what Burgess calls a companionship form of family.

This is probably all very true; in fact it is impossible to believe that in the middle of the twentieth century the structure and function of the family would have remained what it had been in the eighteenth or nineteenth, to look no further back nor further afield than that. Industrialization, the greatest technological advances that man has ever seen, urbanization, the vast increase in knowledge about man and his character and personality—surely it is only to be expected that revolutions of such magnitude would influence the family. But it would be mere romantic longing for the past to assume that things were necessarily better in the good old days, a presumption that seems to underlie much of the discussion of the so-called plight of the American family.

It is not that I am under any illusions that this is the best of all possible worlds. I am as keenly aware as anyone of the festering wounds inflicted by racial and religious prejudice; I know that there are still vast numbers of our population economically deprived, socially outcast, educationally starved, and burdened with numerous other embittering handicaps. What I am trying to establish is a sense of reasonableness and proportion and, indeed, of history in any consideration of family life.

What are supposed to be the symptoms of this widely touted "sickness of American life," about the existence of which there seems to be such agreement? In general these are thought to be: an alarming divorce rate; a staggeringly high incidence of emotional illness; the great increase reported in crime and especially in juvenile delinquency; the high incidence of alcoholism and industrial absenteeism; the persistence of social, racial, and religious prejudice; a value failure and the absence or slowness of our culture advance, especially as indicated by the presumed low taste in American mass activities such as T.V., the movies, etc.; and finally what is thought of as the immaturity or social irresponsibility of the American people. The fact that large numbers of women are employed in industry is not as often viewed with alarm, but the question is apparently still unresolved in the minds of many of the critics of our family life, especially in connection with the imposing rate of divorce and the problem of juvenile delinquency. Also, the lack of religious training and practice is almost always listed as symptomatic of weakness in family life, although perhaps not as often recently as a few years ago. One hears much less of this, although I think there is now some confusion in the interpretation of the figures. An increase in church membership does not necessarily, or even probably, mean there has been a corresponding increase in religious feelings, beliefs, and practices.

Now for myself, I find that I do not view the American family with much alarm, although I recognize that, as any social institution, it is far from perfect. We used to look longingly and admiringly at the primitive who enjoyed freedom from restraint and tension, but we know now that this view was largely illusory and neglected many of the negative (by our standards and values) aspects of primitive social life; we also know that the comparison was not exactly germane. And, too, we used to envy the good old days of big families where grandma or a maiden aunt could baby-sit, and other relatives automatically supplied companionship and "services" within the home. The city dweller envied his country cousins whose family life was so simple, with everything from animals which helped simplify sex instruction to neighborliness which supplied warmth and comradeship, and the collateral family structure with its built-in supports and cohesiveness. (You can live in a city apartment house for years and never know the neighbors who live on the same floor.)

Family life, like other social organizations, is a viable, changing thing as obviously it must be to survive, and it must, in the last analysis, reflect the culture of the country in which it exists, the ethnic nature of its people, their traditions, values, modes of satisfaction, taboos, goals, and ideals. To survive, to flourish, it will reflect these forces and influence them as well. Even in a relatively homogeneous culture this can be a task fraught with difficulties; in a country like our own it is plainly much more difficult to do and indeed to assay.

The anthropologists have reminded us of the dangers of using absolutist standards in judging such a social phenomenon as the family; Benedict especially reminds us how often the family is used as a convenient whipping boy by those who wish to express disapproval of the way the world is going. She emphasizes that it is always necessary to study the family in terms of its fulfillment of its functions in our way of life.

Let us take one or two illustrations from the list of things that have been held, and are still in some measure thought of, as indicative of the "plight" of American family life, and look at them from this perspective.

It has long been held that the fact that a wife, and especially a mother, worked outside of the home was inevitably indicative of tension, conflict, or unfulfilled needs in the home. Except where the catastrophic illness or the death of the husband made it necessary, few "respectable" women worked, and practically none of them in industry. Today married women are able to choose whether and how much they will work; as many as 28 million women were in paid employment in the United States during 1955, accounting for one out of every three workers in the economy. In 1957 they earned a total of 42 billion dollars. Three out of five women who work are married, and about 40 per cent of all mothers in the country with children below the age of 18 are in the labor force. At the turn of the century, half of the women had never worked outside the home and the average work life for all women was about

11 years. Today almost all women work at some time during their lives, and the average young girl can look forward to working at least 25 years. Marriage and children are still the primary goals of today's young woman but, different from last century, she knows she need not forego them to pursue a career or indeed to start to have a career after her children are born and have reached, let us say, their teens. (Here I must again emphasize that these are approximations, applicable essentially to middle-class, largely urban, Americans.)

It is not enough simply to say that this criterion is not valid as an indication of family tensions; I am sure there are many instances where the fact that a mother works does indeed represent tension in the home and, in the most traditional sense, a woman's need or desire to escape. Smuts' recent book on *Women and Work in America* is indeed an effort to "prove" that working mothers are not largely responsible for juvenile delinquency!

It is more helpful perhaps to look on this phenomenon of the woman worker as a reflection of the fluctuation in family life and to avoid a hasty interpretation of its significance. Without attempting at this time any detailed analysis of the shift, we can assume that it reflects not only the social changes that followed the two great wars but also much more complicated and difficult to appraise psychological changes.

In a home where the father's role was automatically presumed to be dominant, even though he was himself not an authoritarian, disciplining person, and the mother's to be passive and compliant, women had no expectation of themselves beyond such compliance and the traditional gratifications of home, kitchen, and children. The girl growing up today is more than likely to have a mother who works at least now and then when some need, personal or perhaps

economic, justifies it; she hears fairly exciting yarns about
her mother's work before marriage and particularly about
her hope and expectation to return to it "when you kids
are a little older." Then, too, her girl friend's mother works,
her aunt is a career woman, and her teacher is married; there
is no longer much fuss about this. While it is certainly true
that the prospects of marriage and children have by far the
greatest importance for the growing girl, the dichotomy
between family and work is no longer quite so clear as it
was; in fact, it is essentially nonexistent. The sequence is
roughly "education, a job, marriage, children, and then I'll
see if I want to go back to work and at what and how
much."

There are, to be sure, family problems which grow out
of the fact that a mother works: feelings of jealousy and
rivalry on the husband's part, often unconscious; distortions
in the child's image of the mother, whose main energies are
not devoted to the care and "service" of the children; tension
in the working mother resulting from the variety of roles
she plays, etc. But, by and large, women and their families
seem to be making this adjustment quite well indeed, and
society too.

To take just one more "symptom" of family tension,
I thought we might look at an equally complicated one, the
divorce rate.

Some years ago two distinguished internists published a
paper in which they accused psychoanalysis of destroying
marriages, and indeed had figures to substantiate this contention. This was and in a measure still is a familiar complaint, and it was true that a large percentage of the people
they had referred to analysts did divorce their spouses,
either during or at the end of their analyses. What they
failed to appreciate was that often the very ability to termi-

nate a destructive, completely unrewarding marriage is itself a sign of recovery (health).

As I mentioned, I have for some time been privileged to
be a consultant at the Arthur Lehman Counseling Service,
where many marital problems come to our attention. Two
things are increasingly apparent to me: one, that I share
with the workers a traditional culture-bound sense of the
worth (if not indeed the necessity) of at least trying to
preserve a given marriage; and second, that divorce rates
are meaningless, considering the high percentage of people
for whom the continuation of marriage is essentially the
perpetuation of the sickest kind of relationship and not in
any sense a socially or psychologically desirable goal.

I would not endorse Benedict's rather cavalier attitude
toward divorce or quite agree with her goals; she emphasizes that the increasing divorce rate is a reflection of the
increased freedom to make marital choices and to change
them, which our culture permits. "Our growing divorce
rate," she says, "is the subject of much viewing-with-alarm;
yet in a culture built as ours is on ever expanding personal
choice, an important goal of which is the pursuit of happiness, the right to terminate an unhappy marriage is the
other side of the coin of which the fair side is the right to
choose one's spouse." It all depends; divorce is often a catastrophic emotional experience for the individual, for children, for the spouse. I know the impressive figures about
the remarriage rate among divorced people, but I also
know the ravages divorce often creates. Here I would
only like to emphasize my belief that it is foolhardy to use
any such isolated criterion as a symbol of the failure of
American family life.

A colleague has recently summed this up very well, saying:

Western civilization has made human dignity, the development of human personality and the inner integrity the center of our concern. These very postulates often lead the individual into conflicts that are insoluble in the traditional way. Marriage counseling, pastoral counseling, and psychiatry are often helpful in removing misunderstandings and clearing up mistakes arising from lack of knowledge, empathy, and sympathy. *But* if the differences in character, upbringing, interests, attitudes, and ethical standards have reached such proportions that they cannot be overcome, no individual can be expected to suffer conditions that prohibit the free expression of his personality and impair his dignity.

There is unfortunately a whole array of still other things for which the family is held responsible. Perhaps the most onerous of these is the incidence of juvenile delinquency, and here we move into the area most difficult and complicated of all. It is certain that what we call juvenile delinquency (and it is, as you realize, an immense assortment of different things variously defined) is increasing—if not at the alarming pace sometimes described, at a great enough rate to challenge all of us who work in the various fields of helping the troubled or who, as citizens, carry the socioeconomic costs of this chaotic phenomenon. We know too that the rates of delinquency are tied to increases in family disruption by divorce, separation, death, or just the sort of family deterioration which has no legal designation but which happens among the socially alienated and economically deprived.

It is clear to all of us who work in whatever capacity with delinquency that it is a most difficult, complicated, and as yet poorly understood problem. If it is unwarranted, as I believe it is, to blame the family for the problems of delinquency, it is no more fair to assume that the family is only a scapegoat. Perhaps it would be best to say it is

the victim of social forces which are disruptive and changing and which bring with them as a consequence such
socially maladaptive phenomena as delinquency. Poverty,
racial and religious prejudice, the high degree of restlessness and mobility in our population, and a general climate
of unrest and disaffection all contribute their share. And,
as recent studies have again emphasized, delinquency is
not a class- or caste-bound phenomenon. To be sure, delinquent behavior looks vastly different in the children of
the economically privileged, but it is in great part quite
the same phenomenon considered from a dynamic point of
view. It is true that in the last analysis the family is the
bulwark against delinquency and that where such behavior
occurs it is usually a family in trouble. It is easy enough
to prescribe love and strength, comfort and control for a
family, but it is infinitely more difficult to know how to
provide these. The "cure" for such problems lies ultimately
in the field of social and economic amelioration, a distant
goal however desirable it may be.

It is tempting to get involved in a fuller discussion of the
delinquency problem but I want to move to some more
general aspects of our subject.

If we assume, as everyone does these days, that the
American family is under special tensions, what are some
of the over-all factors which may contribute to this?

It is usual to begin any such catalogue with some reference to the great tensions arising from the anxiety created
by the threat of atomic warfare. I would be the last to
underestimate the titanic importance of this fact. I can only
say that I am not aware of its effects in the lives of the people I treat or know, and where it is a subject of concern it
seems to be pretty well intellectualized. Perhaps the very
dimensions of the threat are responsible for this; who among
us is really able to cope with the fact that our new radio

telescopes can follow a rocket for a million miles, with measured speeds of over 23,000 miles per hour, or with an announcement that rockets are carefully sterilized to prevent them from infecting the moon? The almost unreal nature of such facts must help us deal with them by denial or by isolation: we come almost to believe "this can't happen to me." At any rate, I must truthfully say that I do not know how to reckon with this factor in the lives of ordinary people. I am not denying that it may very well be an important source of anxiety and tension; I do not know and, frankly, I rather doubt it.

One of the most often cited factors in family tensions is what might be called the restlessness of our people: their failure or inability or lack of opportunity (it may be any of these) to stay put and develop rich roots in an extended family group or a community. Obviously, here too the figures alone are not enough, but they are impressive and should at least be noted. In the United States, from April 1950 to April 1951 (and the trend continues apparently unchanged), over 20 million people (13.9 per cent) moved within the same county, while over 5 million moved within their own state, and a like number were interstate migrants. This represents about 21 per cent of the population. About 35 per cent of all young men in their twenties changed their residence, at an age when so often family life is just beginning.

We are unquestionably a people on the move—restless, curious, and treasuring the very fact of our mobility, as reflected in the highly prized value of "getting somewhere." (Of course, this usually refers to vertical mobility.) After all, this is deeply rooted in our tradition. The old westward movement is proudly remembered in our past, and in our more recent history a vast number of young men and women, through the necessities of war, saw the frontiers of lands of which they had previously not even dreamed. There is no doubt that the earlier extended kinship family group made for a kind of stability and in a way provided its own services: leadership figures, "advice," economic sharing and assistance, baby-sitting and lots else. Goals were set more modestly and values were more deeply rooted.

But even if we assume this to have been highly desirable (and in the narrow terms of family cohesiveness and strength it probably was—or at any rate it looked that way), we must acknowledge that it had to give way before the intensified industrialization of our country; the opening up of newer goals of achievement and success which so often require moving on from one place to another; and of course the shift in the traditional role of the woman in the family. It is not that the newer more isolated family structure is to be preferred; it makes greater demands on the integrity and stability of the individuals involved and robs the family of many of its traditional sources of help and strength. I am sure you realize only too keenly that it is the social agency of one kind or another that has taken over responsibility for the kind of help that was automatically available within the larger family group and long-time neighbors in other days: support in family crises, counseling (advice-giving) of all sorts, economic help in times of need, etc.

I need only mention the mushrooming demand for all the social services in the suburbs of our great cities as a result of their rapid growth. The newly arrived young families look to these services for the help which they can no longer expect from relatives and friends. But I think that while this phenomenon of movement carries certain hazards, it is here to stay; it has indeed become one of our treasured American ways of life—and who would settle for the "good old days" even if he could!

There has been movement in other directions and qualities as well. For instance, there is no question that our overall attitudes toward children and their upbringing have been remarkably revised. A colleague, Martha Wolfenstein, ingeniously studied the bulletins of the U.S. Public Health Service on child rearing over several decades and charted the startling array of changes in the advice offered to parents. For this, psychiatry and psychoanalysis must take much of the responsibility—or, if it turns out that way, the "blame." She demonstrated how indeed our attitudes have become more and more permissive and how this change has contributed to what she called a "fun morality" (a delightfully astute name it is, too). One hears a great deal of invective against this attitude and its presumed corollary, the quest for security, but I wonder if we have not gained as much from this change as we have lost.

In the first place, it represents the inevitable consequence of certain fairly basic social changes: the shorter work week and the great increase in leisure time; the increase in the availability and use of household devices to lighten the woman's burden; the reduction in the father's traditional authoritarian role; and, perhaps most importantly, the basic changes in the child-rearing patterns based on newer psychoanalytic concepts and principles. At worst I would estimate this as a transitory phase in our cultural development, and even here we can perhaps play a role in ameliorating what may be its deleterious features. In a country where free choice exists and "fun" is defined by what people like, I would not be too afraid. Values differ and tastes change; at any rate it is part of an inexorable social process and the final word is far from said about it.

We would be most unhappy if we were presented with a completely static community, incapable of change. It is true that the tempo of the change is fantastic, and there has been little time for adjustment and compromise or the sifting of the good from the negative forces at work in it. But I do not think we need as yet throw up our hands in helplessness or dismay; or that we should fear inevitable doom. Far from it; we have not only greater wealth than ever before but overall a better distribution of it than was ever dreamed of; the opportunity to grow is available to most of the people, as are education and health and welfare services. I realize we still have far to go to a realization of our most cherished goals of equality of opportunity and freedom from want, but we have made a beginning such as would have seemed impossible even a century ago.

As I have said, a greater number now marry, at earlier ages, and have more children. Perhaps a skeptic would say these are not necessarily signs of health in the family structure—or even confidence—but only heedlessness. I would rather think it speaks eloquently for the viability and health of the family, and we may be confident that the institution will persist and survive its current trials and travails. Manifestly this does not mean we must not employ every agency designed to help the troubled family and to prevent social and familial breakdown. This is where the family agencies can play an increasingly vital role. It is for all of us who serve in whatever capacity not to accept glib criticism of the family, but to persevere in our efforts to strengthen and preserve what is good in it—even as we help people and families to grow in ways as yet incompletely understood but great and ennobling in their potential.

III. The Practice of Psychiatry

12. TROUBLED PEOPLE

WE HAVE all of us, I am afraid, begun to weary of the statistics that compel us to face the awful reality that there are by no means enough psychiatrists, psychologists, psychiatric caseworkers, psychiatric clinics, or hospitals. The mere numbers begin now to overwhelm us and, indeed, threaten to paralyze us in a state of hopelessness by their very magnitude. The shortages of trained personnel are estimated in terms of thousands of professionally trained persons—psychiatrists, psychologists, psychiatric social workers, and psychiatric nurses—and tens of thousands of ward attendants and others of more modest training who are needed to help care for the mentally ill and the emotionally disturbed.

These are truly staggering figures; they are just for that reason in a measure unbelievable. The purpose of this paper is to try to make them believable; to bring these statistics alive; to transmute their impersonality and bigness into the story of our neighbors, the little people, the people in trouble.

Some years ago, W. H. wrote this letter to Mary Haworth, a well-known and psychiatrically minded columnist who is widely syndicated throughout the country. Miss

Haworth's column was carried at that time by approximately 150 newspapers in this country and abroad, with an estimated total circulation of ten to twelve million daily.

Dear Mary Haworth:

In my desperation and dark hour I am writing to you in expectation that you may be able to shine the light of hope on my path.

Since October of last year, I have had two nervous breakdowns; and while the first was a terror, the second was worse by far, especially in its tenacity. During this siege I had the services of two fine physicians, but all to no avail. Religion has been sought as a solace, but there again I found only temporary relief.

While I look all right, I am unable to do heavy work and a week ago I lost a temporary job I had and was obliged to let the doctors go, as I can't pay for their services now. Since being out of work this past week, I have sunk into a slough of despair, despite my best efforts to lift myself out. The mental depression gets to be almost more than I can bear at times.

I am a married man and have one child, 20 months old. Because of her, I have carried on. I don't want people pointing their finger at her in years to come, reminding her that her father was a failure and a coward. I am convinced that my difficulty is mental, not physical, and since I am penniless and in need of a psychiatrist, that's why I must appeal to you for help.

It seems I have an obsession—one word has suggested itself to me in my consciousness for years. But since I've been going through this condition, it keeps suggesting itself to me as though some one were whispering in my ear. The effects are devastating to me. The shock is terrific and sometimes I feel as though I were going to lose my mind, which of course I dread. In the name of God, can you help me before it is too late?

W. H.

To which Miss Haworth replied:

Dear W. H.:

Obviously your agony originates in mind. Or, rather, in sub-conscious mind, where lurk the phantoms of all one's child-hood woes that racked the soul with shame and fear, pain and sorrow, and shivering detestation of oneself—to mention just a few of the dread sensations that grip a sensitive child whose sensibilities take a beating in tender years. And I imagine it's no coincidence, your two breakdowns followed close on the heels of fatherhood. I surmise there is a significant connection between the new rôle of responsibility and the uncontrollable outbreak of inexplicable pent-up anxieties you describe.

Perhaps the worry-tension began to mount from the time you married, maybe because subconsciously you ticket your-self a "white sepulcher" sort of fellow who oughtn't and can't afford to get close to anybody, much less undertake the most intimate and responsible human relationships lest your presumption (as you think) or supposed false pretences of being more than you are, lead to shameful defeat of hope and trust, as the test of reality finds you out.

Chronic subconscious antisocial feelings and self-detestation, ingrained in childhood, usually underlie mental outbreaks of terror in later life, such as you suffer now. And psychiatric treatment or psychoanalysis is the road to relief, as you have the good sense to recognize, and as Rabbi Joshua Loth Liebman has made brilliantly clear in his much-discussed book, *Peace of Mind*.

Hence my advice to you, and to others comparably tor-tured, who need psychiatric help, but don't know where to find it nearby—and who can't afford to pay specialist fees—is to write to Dr. George S. Stevenson, Medical Director of The National Committee for Mental Hygiene, New York City, for steering information.

This committee keeps abreast of human developments in the mental health field throughout the whole North American

Continent, from Canada to Mexico, and acts as a clearing house for giving guidance to all who ask.

M. H.

We shall not pause here to consider in any detail Miss Haworth's well-intentioned, but, in the light of present-day circumstances, obviously ill-advised response. Be that as it may, the response to her advice was extraordinary, and well over 2,000 letters were addressed to Dr. Stevenson, as she had directed. Unfortunately, we do not know the exact number of letters that were received. There was no thought of any investigation into these letters at the time they arrived. In many instances they were sent to the various local mental hygiene societies to be answered and we have been able to gather only about 800 of them. Furthermore, in some cities the local newspaper substituted the name of the local mental hygiene society for that of the National Committee, and while we have obtained some of these letters, we do not know how many of them there were. However, this study makes no pretenses to statistical validity; such figures as it introduces are brought in essentially for descriptive purposes. The purpose is to deal with the people rather than with their statistical bulk.

We termed Miss Haworth's response "ill-advised" largely because it held out the promise of a type of direct personal assistance from Dr. Stevenson that could not possibly be forthcoming. But to many of these people, this was also the first inkling they had that there was any help at all for them in their misery. Even more was implicit in this exchange of letters: here was a person who had a position of importance on their local newspaper who calmly accepted the fact of mental illness and was not outraged by it or reduced to moralizing. What Miss Haworth was saying to W. H. was: You have an illness and there are doctors who are trained to treat such illness.

To her readers this acceptance of mental illness and the realization that their own symptoms were not unique to them, or shameful, or beyond help, must have come as a great awakening, and it probably helped many to write so freely of their difficulties.

"I am writing to you for advice. All my life I have been nervous and I had a breakdown in 1929 which lasted six months. I have never had any treatments or advice as I am not able to pay specialists' fees. This is my very first attempt to do anything about it." Or again, "I feel I need psychiatric treatment, but don't know where to turn. Some time ago your address was in our newspaper and I decided to write. Would it be possible for you to put me on the right track?" And yet again: "Not knowing where to turn for advice nor whom to turn to, the article giving your name as reference was most gratefully received. This article said you would help people like myself who cannot afford exorbitant fees to find a psychiatrist. Your help will be appreciated so much."

The secretary of one of the local mental hygiene societies quite understandably comments, after answering many of these letters, "In the back of my mind as I worked on this job I kept thinking that there must be some other way Miss Haworth can make herself useful." Her comment takes on additional poignancy when we read over and over the rather touching dependence of these people on Miss Haworth. ("I read Miss Haworth every day without fail and try always to follow her advice. That's why I'm writing to you now.") We should at least be glad that to many people this column offered a bit of hope and promise that had until then been denied them.

But the thought that "there must be some other way that Miss Haworth can make herself useful" warrants some further reflection. That such widely read and influential

counselors as Miss Haworth, a person already favorably inclined toward psychiatry and with at least a beginning understanding of its functions, could be more properly informed and thus helped to greater service, seems apparent.
I am not in a position to know what efforts have previously
been made to work with her and others; perhaps such attempts have proved impossible. But I do know in what low
esteem such methods of mass communication are generally
held, especially by "us professionals," and how busy we are
in deprecating them. An experience such as this strongly suggests that such columns could be made a most helpful source
of education and suitable advice were it possible to gain the
necessary cooperation on both sides.[1]

What sort of people are these who followed Miss Haworth's advice to write to Dr. Stevenson? In all, we examined 778 letters.[2] The first impression one has of them is the
unexpectedly high degree of literacy, if not always by any
means of knowledge or sophistication, in the writers. Only
rarely—and then practically always from rural areas in the
deep South and in northern New England—did we find the
letter of a borderline illiterate. Again and again the writers
mention that they are high school graduates, and there was
a generous sprinkling of letters from college graduates. Several nurses, a physician, and, indeed, an attendant in a state
hospital were found in this group. The attendant's letter
will perhaps be of interest to you.

I see you quoted quite frequently in Mary Haworth's writing
and that you advise was for the asking. I am nead of some advise on that line. I am 72 years *young* still working but dread-
ing the day I will have to quit. I will more than appricate any
advise you may give me. P.S. I am a night attendant, not a
patient.

The letters were almost all well written, often painfully
frank and revealing, on good stationery, formally correct

as to construction—and so very eager for help. Most often the advice sought was for the writer, but in 232 cases it was nominally for a member of the family, usually a mate, a child, or a friend. Surely in some instances the "friend" is the writer himself, not quite able to face it out, especially in writing. The stigmatization of mental disease is a constantly recurrent theme: "Please answer in a blank envelope as I would not like any one to know I am writing," or, again and again, "any one to know I am mentally sick." In a dozen letters there was the shocking, if not altogether surprising, comment: "I would not like to talk to my doctor about this. In a small town things get around so."

The letters came from forty-five states and Puerto Rico, Newfoundland and Nova Scotia. We grouped them by population of the cities in which the writers live. One hundred and ninety-one, or 26 per cent, lived in cities of over 250,000, and 217, or 29 per cent, in towns of less than 2,500. Both figures are of interest. The former seems quite surprising, since one might have expected a greater degree of knowledge about psychiatry and psychiatric facilities from big city dwellers. A lack of awareness and facilities in small towns was to have been expected.

The writers were predominantly women (75 per cent) and almost 90 per cent were married. The reasons given for writing were basically four: inability to pay standard specialists' fees (26 per cent); dissatisfaction with present treatment (4 per cent); dissatisfaction with past treatment (8 per cent); and, most significantly, lack of knowledge of psychiatric resources (62 per cent).

In only 205 of the letters was it possible to estimate the length of the illness, which ranged from one month to "many years." Twenty-seven per cent of the writers had been ill from one to five years; 30 per cent over five years; and 20 per cent "many years."

I believe it is of considerable interest to review the diagnostic hunches I permitted myself about these people. Obviously these hunches would not bear critical inspection, and I undertook them essentially for one reason. The question would immediately occur to all of us: Are these just crackpots, psychopaths, paranoiacs, and other chronic writers of letters? The opposite proved to be the case. There were only three frankly crackpot letters (one, incidentally, offering, among other things, to start a new mental hygiene society), three letters from dissatisfied patients in state hospitals, and about fifteen from people who seemed paranoid. The rest run the gamut of usual clinical practice: neuroses, marital problems, homosexuality, alcoholism, and psychoses, usually depressions, the last largely in letters grouped as those seeking help for some one other than the writer.

There were a large number of letters (309) requesting merely a list of psychiatrists or psychoanalysts. (In general it can be said that these people have essentially no idea of the distinction. For example, there was the lady who wrote— and on a postcard at that: "My husband is mentally ill and will not go to a specialist and I would like to have him psychoanalyzed without his knowing about it.") Many letters asked for literature. A curious difference in the geographic distribution of those asking for literature was noted, but remains quite unexplained. Massachusetts was not among them.

One interesting aspect of the material was the considerable number of cases in which I thought skilled social casework might well be helpful. Unfortunately, for our purposes, these letters are all quite lengthy, but I venture to reproduce a slightly modified version of one of them to illustrate the type of problem they present.

Dear Sir:

I am very much in need of help an have tried everywhere to get it, but receive the same answer, no matter where I go, so I am writing to you explaining my case in hopes you may be able to help me. As I am getting desperate.

I divorced my husband. I had 2 children by him a boy now 7½ and a girl now 5 years of age. While he was in the service I received support from the Government. Since he has been out of the service he has failed to support them.

I remarried an have a baby girl by him. At the present we are all living at my mothers which is very inconvenient as my mother has old people from the state and we are over-crowded besides that my mother does not want my husband here, which more or less keeps me in a very nervous state. My mother wont send the old people back because this helps her to make ends meet. She says she dont want me or my hus-band, only the children. My two older children do not mind me as my mother has them very much spoiled. Neither my husband or I can correct them without my mother blowing a fuse. She says I was the same. But I cant tell her how hard it is later to be friends with people when you are spoiled. My husband doesn't make enough to buy a home and it is hard to get an apartment with three children. I want to make my older childrens father support them but my husband says he wont let me bring that money in the house even though I say it will help us move.

We tried living with my father in law but he didnt like me or my two children an I took my three children an returned to my mother and finely after being separated for over a month I persuaded my husband to come to my mothers. But living here is just as bad as living at my father in law to add to that my 2 oldest children do not mind.

What I am most interest in is getting support for my 2 children from my first husband. He has been married, divorced and remarried since our divorce. Please help me if you can.

In this same group we should also place the letters from pregnant unmarried girls and also the letters asking for edu-cational and vocational guidance. An especially important group of letters contained requests for marriage counseling, both premarital and later. Many of these letters show fine

insight and emphasize a deplorable lack of information about
the appropriate community agency, even where such exists.

The matter of specialists' fees has now, I imagine, gone
pretty stale. But to these people (166 of them) it was a
matter of primary concern. These letters say, over and over,
"My husband earns about $100 a week and, with children
and all, that doesn't leave much for specialists." Or, "We
could afford five or ten dollars a week, but our doctor says
psychiatrists charge twenty-five dollars a single visit. Where
do decent Christian people like us go?" Or—and this commonly— "We have spent a fortune (for us) on medical care
and injections and now the doctor says we need a psychiatrist. We have only a little left and we hope you can steer
us properly."

A high proportion of all families are only able to save a
few hundred dollars a year, if that. When we realize that
some of these savings had to be put aside for burial insurance, for unexpected medical expenses, and for any number
of other emergency uses, it is clear that the great mass of
the population is in no position to finance for itself even a
minimum amount of psychiatric care.

But money was by no means the only problem. Letter
after letter says, to quote one: "We have money; my husband has a fine farm; not rich, but we'll pay anything. But
as far as we can find out, there are no psychiatrists around
here" (nor, in fact, are there!) "and the doctor is not much
help. He says he doesn't believe in it anyway."

The pattern of a patient seeking help may be graphically
mapped from these letters, and I should chart it as follows:
symptoms; neighborly and family advice; the pastor, except
where the dread of gossip is too strong; the family doctor;
injections and tonics and vitamins; another doctor; a "big"
doctor in a neighboring city; more injections and occasionally gratuitous advice to have a baby, break up a marriage,

give up a job, or whatever, and all the time deepening of symptoms and the growth of hopelessness and despair. No fewer than twenty-five letters inquire, as does this man, "What is left but self-destruction if you can't help me?"—a man who says, "I've been to countless doctors and they all say it's just nerves, and that I've got to get hold of myself"; a man with an overwhelming anxiety state.

Or, as a by-pass on this map—doctors, injections, tonics, vitamins, Christian Science, and then chiropractors. "I thought maybe a chiropractor would help me since the doctor says it's only nerves and they relieve nerves. But even he couldn't help me."

The need for night clinics for people who work, requests for help with children's behavior problems, questions of child adoption and placements, problems reflecting postwar changes and difficulties in adjustment—all these and more were present. Twenty ex-service men and women wrote, in some cases apparently quite unaware of the available facilities provided by the Veterans Administration and, in others, vehemently stating that they would not go to any "army" doctor, no matter what happened.

In another connection [3] I have speculated on the effects on people of the newspaper and magazine publicity about the dreadful state of our mental hospitals. Over and over again we read, "I only know I don't want her [in this instance the writer's wife] to go to a hospital, not after what I've read about them—beating, dirty, bad food, etc. Anything you suggest but that." This is not to deprecate the need for exposing evil where evil exists; I should merely like to note one result of such exposures and one, I think, insufficiently considered in our zeal.

And one could go on, taking almost each and every letter to find a problem in it worthy of our thought and attention. All these letters were answered, but only too often merely to say, "There are no psychiatrists near you"; "You'll have to go a little way across the state line"; "We can well believe you were told you would have to wait six months [six months to a sick person!] before you could be admitted to —Clinic, but there is no other clinic in your part of the state"; all the old, familiar answers.

Let me add still another letter:

Because I'm desperate I'm asking you to help me. I saw your name in a newspaper and I have no one else to turn to. I have feared for years that I was losing my mind and I'm afraid I can't hold on much longer. I have nervous spells and hardly know what I'm doing and feel depressed many days and cry without knowing why. My husband doesn't know what to do either. I feel I will surely lose my mind. I am twenty-three years old and have a three-year-old son and for his sake I don't want to lose my mind.

I have been to many doctors, but none of them have done me any good. They say it is mental trouble. I need a psychiatrist, but every dollar we get has to go for our child, who is not well. Besides, there's no psychiatrist near us and I can't leave and go off anywhere. I'm crazy from worrying about myself. Isn't there any one who can help me?

There is a hell on earth and I'm in it.

These are words spoken for millions. A few lines from letters, a few statistics do no justice to the impact of these pleas. I wish there were some way to share them with you— to fix deep in your memories these fragments of tortured lives. But that is manifestly impossible; instead, I add only my plea to remember, so that we may multiply our efforts, wherever we work, whatever our particular part of the job. In the end, the task is for all of us, and we must not fail those who are in "hell on earth."

13. THE PRIVATE PRACTICE OF PSYCHIATRY

THERE HAS BEEN extraordinary ferment and growth in psychiatry in the past twenty-five years, and it has been my good fortune to participate in and observe the changes that have occurred. It may prove useful to review some of these changes to see which have been fleeting, which more lasting, and to consider some of the lessons to be learned from the changes as well as from those things which have remained steadfastly unchanged. Much of what I shall say will be an extension of earlier comments.[1]

My first teacher in psychiatry was Thomas Salmon. He was genuinely devoted to psychiatry but the curriculum at Columbia allowed him no scope. His reputation rested in good part on his war experience, during which he had been Senior Consultant in Psychiatry for the American Expeditionary Forces. He is still remembered largely for drafting Pershing's cable from France decrying the vast number of emotional misfits who were being sent overseas and demanding that a stop be put to this practice.

My class at school was peculiarly uninterested in psychiatry, and attendance at Salmon's ten or a dozen lectures in the first year was sparse indeed. This was a shame; he was not only a vital teacher but he gave the students in 1920 what was for most if not all of us our first opportunity to hear the magic name of Freud and to learn something of his work. It may be that Salmon, along with others at that time, understood little of what he had read of Freud, but he knew somehow that he had stumbled on greatness and was eager to pass on the word. He encouraged us to read Freud and it was at his suggestion that I began to study the *Introductory Lectures* and *The Interpretation of Dreams*.

There was little else of psychiatry at Columbia in those days to remember. There was not even an independent psychiatric clinic; the patients with emotional and mental problems were seen in the neurology clinic. We were invited to go to the state hospital for a visit in our last year to "see" the patients. I went a few times on my own and was promptly labeled as a freak by my classmates. The paucity of instruction and the official attitude toward psychiatry may well have had something to do with the fact that so far as I know I am one of only two psychiatrists in my class.

I came to Mt. Sinai Hospital as a resident in 1925 and my psychiatric training may properly be said to have begun then. As early as 1913 Oberndorf had organized a psychiatric clinic within the Neurology Department. It was manned by a group of psychoanalytically oriented psychiatrists, even though it had to hide under the title of "Mental Health Class," for respectability's sake! When I came to the hospital, the clinic was headed by Oberndorf and staffed, among others, by such analysts as Lorand, Monroe Meyer, Broadwin, Shoenfeld, and Silverberg. It was a real psychoanalytic treatment and teaching center, the first of its kind I believe in any general hospital in this country.

May I digress at this point to say a word about "Obie," [2] as he has been known to students, colleagues, and friends? I had been at the hospital only a few weeks when a case of hyperthyroidism was admitted to the wards. At that time, these patients were treated by a method euphemistically called "skillful neglect," which consisted of putting the patient to bed, giving him a high caloric diet and plenty of sedation. I had heard casually at medical school that emotional factors occasionally played a role in the etiology of hyperthyroidism, but this remained an academic abstraction until Obie told me to talk to the patient about herself and to listen to anything she wanted to talk about. In 1925 this was revolutionary treatment, and this contrast in the degree of knowledge and sophistication about such matters is one index of the changes that have occurred since. In that instance and in untold others, Obie was a pioneer, enabling me and many others to see the person with the sickness and the life story beyond it, and this before any notoriety had made of psychosomatic medicine an etymological horror and a fashion in medicine.

After completing my analytic training in Europe I began private practice. The alternative to this was a staff job at a state hospital. The opportunities for learning in such hospitals were poor, the salaries inadequate. The demand in the community for psychiatrists was great. Research positions did not exist so far as I knew and I had little, if any, conflict about my choice.

Almost at once I was busy, especially since I was continuing my interest in pathology and holding a part-time fellowship at Mt. Sinai Hospital. I mention my rapidly increasing practice because it posed a problem for me even as it does for young men today. Once one is submerged in an overwhelming load of patients, all plans for study, teaching, and research can quickly evaporate. Then, as now, easy rationalizations were at hand.

My patients fell into two groups, as they have continued to do. There were a considerable number of consultations and a smaller number of patients in therapy. The latter came five or six times a week, and I am a little horrified when my notes reveal clear indications of an unpleasant rigidity about such matters as time and fixity of appointments. Perhaps the first change that struck me as I reviewed early records was the almost total absence of the kind of psychotherapy I now practice a great deal. It is hard for me to remember why it took me some years to apply to private practice the lessons I was learning at the clinic. We saw patients there, as we still do, once or twice a week for about half an hour and the results were often remarkably good. This was and is especially gratifying when one recalls that clinic patients are the least knowledgeable, the most unsophisticated, and, practically without exception, burdened by serious reality problems. I see few patients five times a week, many two or three times, and not a few only once a week. I find this one of the most exciting aspects of practice today as contrasted with my beginning years. It enables me to offer help to a great number who could not possibly afford or manage the time required for intensive therapy.

Of course the debate as to the wisdom of such a procedural change goes on endlessly, and there are still many analysts who see patients only on a five times a week basis. I must say I was heartened when recently I referred a patient to a colleague in another city. I had been seeing the patient two or three times a week in what is now called psychoanalytic psychotherapy, and although she had done quite well, I thought she should undertake more formal analytic work. The patient was ready for this, but my colleague said she saw no one more than three times a week except students in training, and would prefer to continue on this basis with my patient.

The next thing that struck me as I reviewed old records was the almost total shift in the types of illness presented by patients. The most striking changes are these: the manic depressive conditions have practically disappeared from my practice; it has been almost two years since I last saw such a patient. Whereas conversion hysteria, anxiety hysteria, and neurasthenia were frequent diagnoses in the old days, they have been replaced with the obsessive compulsive states, the so-called borderline conditions, and most strikingly, schizophrenia. This is, of course, a purely impressionistic estimate. My experience is not at all uncommon, but we still need carefully controlled studies both to establish the facts of this change and to try to explain it. Obviously it must represent something more than a shift in diagnostic acumen or a change in nosological fashion.

As I reconstruct the situation, I made a diagnosis of schizophrenia with the usual criteria on "typical" patients, almost all of whom I immediately hospitalized. If I saw schizophrenics similar to those I now treat in the office as a routine matter, either they escaped my attention or I labeled them quite differently. Certainly a good number of the then depressions in younger people would be called schizophrenia today. I tested some of these early cases against both my own usual clinical criteria and the Hoch-Polatin criteria for the diagnosis of pseudo-neurotic schizophrenia. In four or five instances I could be certain that a diagnosis of schizophrenia would have been warranted, but there is not the slightest suggestion that I ever thought of such a diagnosis at the time.

More important and much more exciting than this nosological shift is the fact that many of us today treat patients in the office that we would never have dared tackle in the recent past, and with most gratifying results. For myself, practice has outstripped theory, and I use pretty much a homemade sort of supportive, activating, deep therapy which is most difficult to describe, as it is, indeed, to practice, fitting the treatment to each patient in a highly individual way.

One device I find of great help and great interest is that after some schizophrenics, especially the young patients, have reached a reasonable degree of stability, I encourage them to discontinue office treatment but to remain in close touch with me by letter and telephone. This has its drawbacks; my wife has come to know the inevitable evening calls and to recognize Tom or Mary. Her comment is that she thinks I am doing first rate casework with these patients, a compliment perhaps of some theoretic interest.

Many patients I see now are in the general range of character disturbances; people who are having difficulties in interpersonal relations but with few if any "symptoms." They work, often at top level jobs; they function in society, often quite usefully from society's point of view; they are on boards and committees and belong to organizations but withal they are miserable. It is certainly tempting to reflect on their illness as part of our world's tensions. But I am not fully persuaded. It seems reasonable to expect that these tensions contribute to our patients' difficulties, but I wonder if they do more than provide the setting within which the illness develops.

Then there are many patients with psychosomatic problems, who are referred because they suffer from illnesses in which emotional factors are now clearly recognized. There are two interesting extremes in these patients as I see them—they usually are referred too early or (and this is clearer) much too late. I see a steady stream of patients referred by doctors who work in highly sophisticated hospital settings. These patients have relatively minor symptoms but are told that these are manifestations of emotional illness and that they should seek analytic help.

My favorite illustration of this group had been a young

man who was referred to me because of a single patch of psoriasis, but recently I saw an equally impressive example of "premature" referral. A young man, an applicant for a position requiring a preliminary physical examination, fainted when blood was drawn from a vein. He told the examining physician of one similar incident while in the Army. He is in excellent health, happily married, has good relations with his children, has had excellent and satisfying jobs, and is in line for promotion to a top executive post.

Theoretically one might say that in each case there was a symptom which suggested, or in the instance of the man who fainted, indicated an emotional conflict. Both of the referring physicians have real knowledge of psychodynamics and one of them has had a successful therapeutic analysis. But weighing the symptom against time, money, and lack of motivation, I advised the patient not to start an analysis. The physician of the man who fainted disagreed with me and sent the patient to another analyst who undertook therapy with him. The internist, a close friend, reported that my colleague attributed my opinion less to a lack of knowledge of pathology than to my general "conservatism"!

The rightness of my estimate is not important; I wonder if we have not become overly sensitive to the role of emotional factors in illness, and if especially in our teaching of undergraduates, we are not a bit too enthusiastic and somewhat unrealistic. One therapeutic tool is available for such patients and too infrequently used. In the clinic we often get satisfying results from casual, supportive psychotherapy in many psychosomatic problems, but confronted with similar problems in private practice, we seem impelled to offer intensive, reconstructive therapy or nothing. This is rather a shame; I know no more grateful patients than those freed from a distressing symptom even though nothing more profound is attempted. I recently saw a man of fifty with a lifelong character problem and anxiety state. He had finally developed frightening and crippling attacks of angina-like pain. It was possible for him to come only once a week, and in twenty-odd sessions his pain had gone, although to be sure he was still the same rigid, domineering, egocentric character. I do not think this any miracle but only a satisfactory result of therapy based on the limited and realistic goals which I had set for both the patient and myself.

But as though to negate my conservatism and undo my caution, I must say that most of the patients I see with somatic illness have been far too long coming to a psychotherapist. Two illustrations: A forty-nine year old man, tense, overactive, overambitious, had frank overt symptoms of colitis for eleven years. He had had innumerable proctoscopies and X-ray examinations, and one laparotomy in which only his appendix was removed, but which he was led to believe would result in a shunting of the food past the diseased bowel. On his doctor's advice, he had taken two leaves of absence, each lasting a year or more, and was finally referred to me by a urologist whom he had consulted not about colitis but about his diminishing sexual potency. When asked by the patient if he should undertake analysis, his family doctor said, "I never knew a sane analyst in my thirty years of practice but if you want to go to one, that's your funeral." I must report not only that the patient is persistently ill as the result of a severely scarred and deformed lower bowel, but that eleven years of extraordinary secondary gains from illness make it difficult to effect a real change. Recently, his doctor made a home visit to see the patient's wife for some minor illness and paid the patient (and me) a minimal compliment by saying: "You must be better. At least you waited until morning to call me instead of your usual call at 2 A.M."

A young man was referred to me by an internist who had recognized the nature of the patient's asthma and told him bluntly that he needed psychotherapy. The patient was passive, dependent, tense, and self-deprecating. Every escape from home and mother was blocked by illness which forced him back, literally, to his mother's home, though he was obviously never far from it psychologically. He needed and wanted psychological help but was for years dissuaded by his family doctor who told him that he would be wasting his time and money, and that he (the doctor) had never seen a patient helped by psychoanalysis. This doctor, by the way, suffers from lifelong, severe, and debilitating migraine!

When I began in practice, psychoanalysis and psychiatry were quite suspect, and the doctors with whom I was associated were often critical, suspicious, and questioning, and referred patients in a manner that seemed to say, "All right, show me what you can do." I remember bitter conferences, tense ward rounds when psychoanalysis was openly mocked, and certain chiefs who referred only "hopeless" cases for psychiatric consultation.

It was clear that one of my greatest responsibilities as a private practitioner would be a kind of public relations-educational-liaison job with the referring doctors. I still believe it but if we have gained a vastly greater acceptance of our work, it is hardly because we deal more adequately with the general practitioner or specialists who send us our patients. In my opinion, we hide behind the obvious necessity for observing our patient's confidences to disregard the physician, to treat him with scant courtesy and often with deprecating condescension.

Just one example of this: A physician, a close friend, referred a patient to me following her return home after a profound psychotic depression requiring hospitalization. For three years I saw her on a casual basis and not entirely satisfactorily. I finally suggested she undertake an analysis and recommended a consultation. She went to see the consultant of my choice who sent her to a younger analyst without ever discussing this with her doctor or me. When a change to still another analyst was necessary, we were neither of us asked about the wisdom of the move or the choice of person. Now, I am not speaking of people at the periphery of our profession but of trained, experienced people of repute. What does one do when a highly reputable and experienced medical colleague, a great admirer of the psychiatric skills, tells one that with rare exception he has never had a report from any analyst to whom he has referred a patient, rarely even a courtesy note or call to thank him for the referral, and that in general he assumes he no longer has any relationship with patient or analyst, once therapy has begun. I would be more eager to question these yarns or ascribe them to jealousy, if my own experience with analysts to whom I refer patients was not essentially identical. When I send a patient to an analyst, I ask him to please let the referring doctor know that the patient is in therapy, perhaps give him a notion as to the diagnosis and possible prognosis, and once in a while perhaps drop him a line telling him what goes on. I can only say this is rarely done: in fact I have had patients referred to other analysts by the person to whom I sent them so that I am unable to tell the referring doctor who is treating his patient. When a friend tells me that with very few exceptions he finds he no longer takes care of the medical problems of his patients who are in analysis, I cannot believe this reflects only his own attitudes and it surely cannot reflect on his competence and skills, which are outstanding. I believe this is worse

today because analytic time is difficult to arrange and the
general attitude seems to be that the analyst is doing the referring physician a favor.

Looking through my early records naturally brought me
to some reflections on the cost of my services and of psychiatric services in general. In a city like New York our
skills and talents are available to a very small degree to the
poor who attend clinics and almost entirely to the economically upper classes whom we see in our offices. (The
only exceptions to this are a group of professional workers,
especially social workers, who seek and get analytic help
but often at a cost which impoverishes them and robs them
of even some necessities for reasonably decent living. They
often seek such help for minimal problems and can rarely
be induced to undertake anything but "classic" analysis.
There are many unresolved questions about this group of
people.)

In general, if one accepts as a minimal fee fifteen dollars a session and three times a week as a minimal requirement, we have an expense of over two thousand dollars a
year, a staggering sum, and out of reach of any except a
tiny percentage of the population.[3] I understand this, more
or less, but I contend that it is very difficult to do one's
work responsibly under such socially deleterious circumstances. This is a value problem of the first order and unless
we can find methods to deal with it, I believe it must en-
danger our work. From candidate selection, through training, and on to practice, we are encouraging a tendency
which I believe should be scrutinized critically. Aside from
the painful impact it may have on an individual patient in
quest of help, it has even more important *social* significance
and consequences.

Another aspect of private practice that I regret to find
has not improved is the problem of the patient who needs

to be hospitalized. Here again, the cost is a serious deterrent to prompt and proper referral; the inadequacies of care in all except one or two hospitals present a discouraging picture; and the still complete disregard for the referring psychiatrist is for me at least a source of annoyance and often embarrassment. The father of a schizophrenic girl I had referred to one of the oldest and reputedly best private mental hospitals in our vicinity called to ask when I wanted to see the girl now that she was home. I referred her to this hospital nineteen months previously. In that time, I had a note telling me she had been admitted and asking for a summary of my experience with her, a copy of a standard status sent on my special request and no further word of any kind at any time whatsoever. I visited her twice because of the family's insistence: I avoid such trips since they usually serve only to satisfy the family's need for information which could and should be given by the staff.

The introduction of shock therapies represents the most noticeable and dramatic change in practice through the years.[4] I remember with remarkable vividness the night we saw the first patient who had improved with insulin shock therapy. She was an old catatonic schizophrenic, in such a deteriorated condition that it was thought "safe" to treat her. And to be sure, she had "improved" in that she would now get out of bed and managed to make sounds that were more or less intelligible. I recall even more vividly Jelliffe's brilliant discussion of the great day ahead in which schizophrenics would be cured promptly and certainly with this new magic. Only those who knew Jelliffe can understand the excitement of the evening and the illusions we carted home with us.

I have no statistics and they would not be reliable; I can only say that with few exceptions I find the use of the various forms of shock therapy most disappointing in practice.

The postpartum depressions of which I see few since they are usually referred directly to psychiatrists (and nonpsychiatrists) who do shock therapy; the depressions at the menopause which, for the same reason, I rarely see in practice, and the depressions of the later years do well with electric shock therapy, but that would about end my list. In schizophrenia, except where intense excitement occurs, I prefer the tools of psychotherapy. One of my friends, an enthusiast for shock therapy, complains he has the worst luck just with *my* patients.

There is a climate to private practice. How does it differ from that which existed when I began in practice? First, there is much more acceptance of our work at all levels—patients, families, physicians, other professions, social agencies, universities. It is rare these days for a lay person, much less a physician, to ask that I see an unwilling patient and tell him I am a "nerve specialist" but to be sure not to mention that I am a psychiatrist.

Of course, there are those who hold that we have gone to the other extreme in publicizing our work. I doubt that. It is true that among certain groups there is a special distinction in having been analyzed. Occasionally one trembles at news which comes out of certain gatherings such as the recent Parent-Teacher Association meeting where a psychoanalyst told the audience that every parent should be analyzed if he or she wanted to do the "best possible job" with their children.

The climate of private practice is unsettled by such wranglings in the press as the perennial fight about the practice of psychotherapy by nonmedical persons. There are few things that the laity knows less about than the so-called "schools" of psychoanalysis, but their concern with the subject seems great. As the psychiatric-psychological self-help books pour from the press, I find myself increasingly taxed to get patients to tell me what they feel and not what they think this or that means. This was not a problem twenty-five years ago and I truly believe the patients were better off for their very lack of "knowledge."

I find my patients not as concerned as I would expect with world issues nor is this so far as I can discern a reflection of particular pathology. It is by no means only the withdrawn schizoid type of patient who is apparently untouched by these tensions. Even the announcement of the H-bomb and the test that apparently got out of hand did not stir up the anxiety I had anticipated. I know that the world of the neurotic reflects special fears but it is still startling to watch the preoccupation with trivia persist even in the face of world shattering events. Certainly these events produce nothing like the panic the stock market produced in my patients, itself a sad commentary on our world.

What of results? It is now an ancient truism that we need to know much more about our results but nothing much is done about it. I have just been over the records of all the patients I have had in therapy. I tackle patients now whom I would never have treated in the office earlier, but I do not believe that this reflects any growth in technical knowledge. It rather represents my experience, a more secure place in the profession, and a greater willingness to assume responsibility. By rule of thumb, from experience, from scrutiny of my failures as well as my successes, I have made many shifts in technique, such as I believe every one makes after years of practice. I find little opportunity for *direct* application of our greater theoretical knowledge; it helps me in my own understanding of the dynamics but I do not see direct connections between the advances in theory and the kind of loosely structured methods I follow.

I believe my results are now generally better, an improvement stemming from several things: (1) more modest goals after a period when as a result of newly developing theory, especially around the greater understanding of ego function, I was too ambitious and perfectionistic in my goals; (2) the practice of trial periods of intermission in the work; Oberndorf emphasized this years ago but it is only in the last five years or so that I have fully explored the merits of this technical device; (3) starting with very sick patients, I am free to interpret as improvement, relative changes toward health which might not be as clearly discernible in less sick patients.

I have left for the last what I consider to be the greatest and in some ways the most important change in my practice and that is my relation to the community. When I began, practice was indeed a "private" matter with only the hours spent in the clinic and hospital as interludes. Like most psychiatrists, I now play an every increasing role in community affairs. We are involved in education, services to social and other community organizations, and research. The role of the psychiatrist in interdisciplinary research is a significant and important recent development.

There are no limits now to the vista of opportunities to work with people in a whole array of nonclinical settings both as teacher and as advisor. Although I do a fair share of such educational work, candor requires me to acknowledge that I am still not entirely persuaded of the wisdom of much that is done in this field, and I feel most emphatically that we need to know much more about the effects of our efforts than we now do before we can be certain that we are really accomplishing our goals.

14. PSYCHIATRIC CLINIC PRACTICE *

THE TREMENDOUS dearth in psychiatric personnel and facilities became apparent very early during World War II. This was no novel observation; those of us who had worked in psychiatric clinics knew that they were understaffed and that resources for adequate care of ambulatory patients with psychiatric problems were shockingly deficient. However, it took the war situation with its appalling number of neuropsychiatric rejectees and, as the war progressed, of psychiatric dischargees, to bring the lack to sharper awareness.

In reports such as the one issued by the New York City Committee on Mental Hygiene,[1] it was pointed out that approximately three quarters of the neuropsychiatric rejectees and dischargees in New York City were without psychiatric help of any kind, private or public. Over and over again the call was made for more psychiatrists, psychiatric social workers, and psychologists; various estimates, such as Lawrence Kubie's [2] of 21,000 psychiatrists, have become so familiar as to form a cliché in our thinking about the problem. Hence the preoccupation with this obvious, if immensely important, fact. We have almost spun the illusion that this lack is the sole factor in the inadequacy of

* Written with Winifred Arrington, M.S.S.

facilities. Granting the lack, it seemed the more imperative that we seek for other factors which might possibly be involved, lest we remain enmeshed in the discouraging helplessness that contemplation seems to induce.

The New York City Committee on Mental Hygiene has long been interested in psychiatric clinics as part of its larger concern with the mental hygiene problems of the community. Accordingly, it undertook a study of clinic facilities primarily designed to study the efficacy of the use of clinic time. It is surprising to find how little attention has been given, at least in published studies, to psychiatric clinic practice, although this obviously represents an important part of the over-all psychiatric problem. In general, speculations about psychiatric care focus on the efficacy of particular treatment methods in definite clinical situations, weighing one against another. This is certainly a valid enough approach, but we [3] decided against using it as the focus of this study for various reasons. Most important was our desire to try to establish criteria which would permit the possibility of a more objective estimate than the weighing of therapeutic results which are notoriously difficult to control and evaluate. Perhaps as important was the fact that a large part of clinic time is devoted to functions which cannot be considered therapeutic at all, but which use a great deal of the available service.

The details of the methodology are not essential to this presentation. This analysis deals with but a few of the insights gained from the study and with reflections growing out of the authors' experience in psychiatric clinics.

Four psychiatric clinics were chosen for study representing, so far as external circumstances permitted, contrasting types of clinics found in New York City. These clinics are designated by letters, not so much in the hope or expectation of disguising their identity, but rather to emphasize that

these remarks are not to be construed as critical of the clinics
or their personnel. We acknowledge the splendid cooperation we enjoyed throughout from the directors and staffs
of all the cooperating clinics.

The procedure used was a simple one. In three of the
four clinics, records of all the patients seen during a two-
month period were read and abstracted in detail by the
social workers. In the fourth clinic, which is much smaller,
the records for the entire year were read in order to obtain
a comparable sample. The cases were drawn from clinics
whose personnel had been sharply reduced by the war
situation, and every effort was made to allow for this factor
in the interpretation of the findings.

The findings were recorded in the greatest detail on a
form devised for this purpose. The cases were divided into
two major classes—treatment and advisory. Actually, four
types of services were recognized: *consultation* cases, in
which the clinic undertakes to offer advice or steering as
well as diagnosis, and assists referring agencies in carrying
out plans for the patient; *teaching* cases (three clinics carried a responsibility for teaching undergraduates, although
in one instance that assignment had been allowed to go
largely by default because of the lack of personnel); *treatment* cases, in which the clinic plans to offer some form of
psychiatric treatment to the patient; and, finally, there were
cases accepted primarily for *research*. Obviously these functions overlap in some instances and such cases were classified in accordance with the major emphasis.

It must be remembered that this work has been based
entirely on records and that we had no contact with patients except through their records and interviews with
their doctors and social workers. Having digested the case
thoroughly, the worker attempted an estimate of success-

ful and unsuccessful use of clinic time in terms of service to the patient. The following summarizes the criteria used in the scoring.

1. Advisory Service

Effective advisory service may be considered rendered if any of the following is represented.

a) Diagnostic report is given *to the patient* who (in reader's judgment) is capable of using the information constructively. Opportunity for discussion of the report is also given.

b) Diagnostic report and opportunity for discussion is given *to a relative* when circumstances warrant, and the relative is able to make constructive use of the information.

c) Diagnostic report is given *to an agency* which has assumed responsibility for helping the patient with his problems.

d) An explanation is given *to the patient* who is capable of using it constructively. Explanation is given in place of a diagnostic report but is designed to help the patient understand and accept his condition, when indicated, and possibly plan his future course.

e) An explanation is given *to a relative* who can use it constructively on behalf of a patient who cannot. Based on diagnostic data, this explanation is such as to help the family understand and accept the patient's condition and make effective plans for him.

f) Consultation service given to responsible agency or clinic is directed toward helping the agency relate diagnosis to planning.

g) Any valid advisory service not included above.

2. Treatment

a) Social or vocational improvement: The patient is able, following treatment, to enter into social or work activities previously impossible, or is better able to function in his environment. There must be real evidence of this in the record as, for example, the report of a better job, recognition in the form of more pay or responsibility, ability to make new friends, etc.

b) Symptomatic improvement: The clinic succeeds in creating in the patient better *tolerance* for his symptoms, or helps him to see that adaptations in his living arrangements will lessen irritation from his symptoms. Treatment results in the *modification* or *disappearance* of the patient's symptoms. The patient is able to *perceive* for himself the relationship between his behavior or attitudes and his underlying feelings. The term *recovery* is used in its usual clinical sense. *Other* means any positive outcome of treatment.

Each research record was then reviewed by the psychiatrist and, in case of doubt as to the proper scoring, he also read the original clinic record. Finally, each case was discussed at a staff conference and all points of variance reconciled.

At this point we should like to digress briefly to discuss the matter of records. Social work rightly devotes a great deal of time and attention to the recording process; so far as we know, no psychiatrist has ever been so instructed. To put the matter quite bluntly, the records in these clinics and, we are sure, in others as well, reflect this. Granting all the factors of time and the pressure of work, the records failed in almost all instances to give any adequate idea of the problem involved, the therapeutic goal, the rationale of the particular approach that was utilized, the reasons for decisions, such as changes in therapists, referrals for psychological and other examinations, reasons for termination or at least some speculation about it, and so on. In 76 per cent of all treatment cases and 94 per cent of all advisory cases the reason for termination is not stated. Nor was a diagnosis advanced in any but a few cases except in one clinic (Clinic C), where every case has a tentative diagnosis noted in the record of the admission interview.

Aside from purposes of research where records such as these are strikingly barren, it must surely remain a matter of great question if the resources of a clinic are fully utilized even in the direct task of caring for patients so long as their records remain chaotic. Certainly the entire question of recording needs to be critically reexamined.

In the final analyzed sample of 288 cases, 150 were treatment cases and 138 advisory. The study of these cases affords many significant findings of which, for lack of space, we discuss only two. The first concerns a factor in psychiatric clinic practice which we consider of the first importance. Though recognized by people working in psychiatric clinics, it has thus far had scant critical attention. Our own interest in this particular problem dates from an earlier study, in which was found that of 1,185 men rejected or discharged from the armed services for neuropsychiatric reasons and referred to appropriate treatment facilities, 676 visited the clinic one to three times; of these, 385 appeared once. It could be said even by the most generous estimate that only 291, or less than 25 per cent, were ever really under psychiatric care.[4]

So striking a phenomenon, representing as it does an immense waste in the use of psychiatric resources, obviously demanded further scrutiny beyond what was possible in that particular study. Why do so many patients who present themselves for treatment fail to return to the clinic? More and perhaps clearer evidence on this point may be available on the completion of a further study in which it is hoped to interview such patients in their homes. We feel, however, that evidence already available casts considerable light on this complicated problem.

We were not surprised to learn that of the patients here reported, over one third (38 per cent) dropped out before the fifth visit. This constituted 47 per cent of all cases that were judged "unsuccessful" since no effective service had been rendered them.

The first factor to be considered, and probably one of the most important, is the influence of the referral process. How adequately has the patient been prepared for the referral to a psychiatric resource? How well does he understand its purpose and limitations? Of the treatment cases, 50 per cent understood more or less that they were coming to the clinic for treatment of an emotional problem; 17 per cent had no personal reason for accepting the referral; and 13 per cent came for some vague, undefined help. In other words, in the latter cases the reasons for referral were probably improperly explained to the patient or he was not ready at that time to use referral to a psychiatric facility.

Other factors were discovered in the analysis of the records of those who discontinued treatment. The "last" visit was studied separately; thus, if a patient dropped out after his second visit, the experiences of all patients on second visit were tested to find which factors resulted in discontinuance of treatment. Then the first five visits of patients were considered together. Thus, we sought an answer to the question—if a certain event occurs during early clinic experience, does it tend to create resistance to continue?

A number of contributing factors were discovered. For instance, if patients were asked to confer with a new person after the first visit, the percentage of those who failed to return was markedly increased; similarly, if confronted with more than one "doctor" (the quotation marks are designed to include medical students, "doctors" in our medical tradition!) after the first visit. If this is to be interpreted as reflecting discomfiture, or hostility to the lack of privacy and to the impersonality of seeing several doctors at once, we are left with a seeming paradox for which we have no ready explanation. When patients were asked to see more than one person on their very first visit to the psychiatric clinic, no such increase in discontinuance was found. Curiously enough, what happened during a patient's first visit to the clinic played a seemingly unimportant role in determining "dropping out" in a particular case. Otherwise this finding is in accord with our general observation that where patients were required to consult with more than one representative of the clinic (psychiatrist and psychiatric social worker or psychiatrist and psychologist, etc.) *during a given visit to the clinic,* the effective rate, by the standards of our research, was very low (7 per cent compared with a high of 50 per cent). Repeated and fairly formal psychiatric examination and history-taking seemed to increase discontinuance; this usually resulted from shifts in student groups and the assignment of a new student psychiatrist.

Considering all the patients' visits as a group, additional factors were discovered. It is not surprising that early contact with a social worker made for a distinct advantage; more than twice as many patients who saw a psychiatric social worker during their first four visits continued in treatment (45 per cent as compared with 21 per cent).

In contrast to this were the clinics' policies so far as their use of social workers is concerned. Only in Clinic D were practically all the patients seen by a social worker before being seen by the psychiatrist. In Clinic A it may be fairly stated that no social work was done at all. In Clinic B the functions of the social worker were in good part administrative and supervisory, and she saw only an occasional patient for casework service. In Clinic C a social worker saw patients on special request of the psychiatrist but so far as this series of cases is concerned, we found few where the caseworker's skills were so engaged. However, in this clinic workers did participate actively in the teaching of medical students. Granting full weight to certain external pressures implicit in the war setting, we found little integration of casework in the function of these four clinics. In Clinic D, for instance, there was but one worker and, by her own statement, her job was not a "casework job." It was estimated by the staff that at least three of four workers would be necessary to do even a tolerably adequate job.

There is one other factor to be mentioned. Where a relative of the patient visited during the first five visits, the percentage of discontinuance was almost halved; 43 per cent dropping out where no such visit occurred, 25 per cent where a relative did visit.

To summarize: the discontinuance of patients before the fifth clinic visit represents an immense waste of clinic facilities. Such patients represent almost half of those whose attendance resulted in unsuccessful use of clinic time, and a comparable proportion of the clinic's available service is thus wasted. Factors of poor referral, inadequate preparation, and invasion of the privacy of the doctor-patient relationship all make for such termination. On the other hand, the use of social workers, calling the family into the clinic relationship, and an understanding by the patient of the function of the psychiatric referral militate against the early termination of the patient's contact with the clinic.

We now shift to the consideration of a quite different aspect of clinic practice. This divergence is occasioned by the necessity for reasons of time to limit ourselves to but two major aspects of the question of psychiatric clinic practice.

For some time there has been, and rightly so, a tremendous ferment in psychiatric education at all levels, including the undergraduate. Those who are responsible for policy are understandably concerned with the reexamination of the goals and functions of such instruction. Psychiatric outpatient departments are used for the education of medical students by a number of medical schools, and we should like to turn our attention to some aspects of this problem which we believe have been illuminated in the course of this investigation.

As already mentioned, one of our four clinics (D) carried no teaching responsibility whatever, and another (A) had practically been compelled to allow its teaching function to go by default during the time covered by this study, mainly because of an extreme shortage of personnel. Our observations on this subject are therefore confined largely to two clinics.

In Clinic C fourth year students were assigned, approximately ten at a time, for four sessions weekly, each lasting three hours and continuing for one month, or a total of 48 hours. Of this time, one hour of each session was allotted to a lecture, two half-hour periods to work with the supervising psychiatrist, leaving one hour during which the student saw a patient. Allowing, as was customary, one visit a week for a patient, this permitted the student to see a given patient a maximum of four times and usually enabled him to see four patients.

The stated aims of teaching in this clinic were described as follows: to give the student an appreciation of an ambulatory psychiatric patient and to give him awareness of mental and emotional symptoms and their meaning.

Each session was divided so that the student, as one of a group of three or four, spent a half hour with a supervising psychiatrist to discuss general problems of interviewing, saw his patient for approximately an hour, and then had another half hour with the supervising psychiatrist, this time individually, to discuss the interview he had just had. Occasionally student and supervisor saw a patient together, but patients in this clinic were never seen by groups of doctors.

At Clinic B the students were in the third year of medical school and were assigned to the psychiatric clinic for three months. During this time they had two sessions each week of approximately two hours each and one conference each week. Hence, they were allotted a total of 48 hours with patients and twelve conference hours during the three months. It should be noted that the assignment to the psychiatric clinic represented, for one group in each class, the students' first contact with patients. Each student was expected to see patients in seven diagnostic categories (depression, schizophrenia, hysteria, behavior problems of childhood, organic syndrome as seen in senility, a psychosomatic case such as colitis, ulcer, etc., and a case of feeblemindedness).

A great deal of the ultimate responsibility in this clinic for the teaching method was given to the individual instructor ("each instructor is his own boss"), hence various teaching techniques were employed. The patient might be interviewed by the instructor with one or more students "listening in" (the number might be as many as five); the patient might be interviewed by the student alone. One such interview was necessary as each student must submit a "mental status" as part of the requirements for the completion of the course. The patients' appointments were made at various intervals, weekly, biweekly, etc., to insure the student a suitable variety of cases. Occasionally, but rarely, a conference with the social worker was requested by the instructor in which the student participated.

Here are two quite obviously divergent concepts of teaching, though the differences are perhaps not as striking as appear on the surface. In Clinic C an attempt is made to enable the student to work with one patient during the four weeks he attends the clinic. This accomplishes a nominal continuity of endeavor, and from this point of view may represent some advantage. It will shock no one, we are sure, that a careful reading of the records at this clinic fails to reveal on the student's part any substantial concept of the basic problems involved, the dynamic considerations, etc. Even a seasoned psychiatrist would more often than not be baffled by the complexities of many of these patients' problems and not consider it at all amazing that four sessions with a patient had failed to make either much therapeutic progress or given the therapist an entirely adequate concept of the dynamic situation.

The question is frequently asked: Does the teaching process "harm" the patient? This is difficult to decide; in terms of really discernible injury to the patient, our study, so far as it went, failed to reveal evidence of any such harm. Where the students' participation could be separated out (and this was possible really only in Clinic C), students were solicitous, kindly, interested in the patients' problems, and comforting. It should be noted here that by our criteria, visits with medical students had the highest effective rate. This would suggest that the students' avidity and interest and concern with the patients' actual problems had a most salutary effect.

At Clinic B the emphasis is entirely on the teaching material and the therapeutic effort falls largely on the instructor. The consideration of a "beautiful treatment case" is of first importance. In both clinics relatively little is known of the new patient at the point at which the student sees him, and little consideration can be given to possible attitudes and feelings on the patient's part in regard to his examination by a student. At Clinic C cases for the students are chosen largely from among those long in attendance at other clinics, and hence quite well inured to clinic processes and usually fairly well "somaticized" in their own estimates of their illness.

At Clinic B the emphasis is on exposure of the student to an abundant variety of clinical material; at Clinic C a more conscious and deliberate effort is made to give the students at least a beginning awareness of the meaning of the patient's symptoms and their relation to his total life situation, with much less concern about the number of diagnostically different types of illness to which the student may be exposed.

As to the question of what student psychotherapy accomplishes or fails to accomplish, the evidence is not at all clear. The director of Clinic B stated he was sure that the patients' gain from what is done in the interests of teaching outweighs any harmful effects; on the other hand, the director of Clinic C thought it necessary to select patients who were insensitive enough or confirmed enough in their difficulties to be relatively unaffected by anything which the student might or might not do.

The influence of teaching on the selection of patients is

most important. At Clinic B there is no mistaking the fact that the interests of the student take precedence over the interests of the patient, and, to a considerable extent, clinic intake is governed by the interests of the teaching program. As indicated above, the teaching plan in this clinic is designed to give the student contact with seven major diagnostic groups, and the teaching staff keeps a list for each student to make certain that he has seen at least one patient in each of the seven groups. It is impossible to escape the implications of this plan. In order to provide every student with at least one of seven different types of patient, the clinic must admit a sufficient proportion in each of these diagnostic groups to keep the supply adequate. Since three of the seven selected groupings are hardly ideal for clinic treatment, one can assume that a considerable proportion of clinic intake must be made up of nontreatable patients or those for whom treatment offers small promise of success.

In the case of Clinic C, reference has already been made to the fact that the attempt is at least made to assign to students patients who are not likely to be damaged by amateur handling and frequent shifts of interviewers. The chronic or medically conditioned patient is more often selected for student purposes, and the more hopeful and actually treatable patient is, so far as possible, referred to other persons on the clinic staff than those engaged in teaching or learning. The relative proportion of the latter to the former within total clinic intake, however, is kept low by the small number of "treatment psychiatrists" on the staff and the relatively high number of teaching psychiatrists and students.

Teaching also influences the frequency of contact of the patient with the clinic. At Clinic B more than one interview is possible in given cases for purposes of initial inquiry and examination, but thereafter the frequency of the student's contact with the patient is determined as much by the exigencies of the student's own program (such as his need to be scheduled for appointment with patients in six other diagnostic categories) as by the status of the patient's problem and his need for supportive or other therapy. This may mean that regardless of the patient's need for early renewal of the contact, interviews may be scheduled two weeks apart or at even longer intervals. It is assumed, of course, that spacing of interviews will take as much account as possible of both sets of interests, but practically speaking, the requirements of the teaching schedule are quite capable of interfering with the treatment needs of the patient.

At Clinic C the scheduling of patients' interviews is, on the whole, quite systematic. The length of the individual student's stay in the clinic is limited to four weeks and the teaching plan requires that the same patient be seen on the same day of each week by the same student. This, therefore, means a maximum of four interviews which any given patient will have with any given student. There is, however, an implied promise to the patient in that, theoretically, if he wishes, a certain hour of a certain day remains his during the term of the student whom he is currently seeing; the hour can continue to be his in later weeks with a series of succeeding students. It is true that later appointments may be scheduled two weeks apart if the patient's improvement or lack of improvement suggests less need.

It is clear that the clinic program is alone among the teaching services under discussion in guaranteeing to the patient privacy of interviewing. It arranges for all discussion about the patient, either between the student and his supervisor or between the supervisor and a group of students, to take place in the patient's absence.

At Clinic B, privacy of interviewing is possible on occasion but is seldom practiced. It would appear here that the only real provisions for a student's seeing a patient privately occurs when the student is having his required experience doing a "mental status." There are certain other possibilities for private interviewing, but from all indications they are infrequent rather than routine. Each student is expected to see one new or continuing patient every time he is in the clinic. Although he may, in some instances, see his patient alone, he is more likely to see him in the presence of one to five other persons. These additional persons include, in addition to the teaching psychiatrist, one or more of his fellow students.

On the basis of contact with the teaching procedures of the clinic, we were able to construct a partial definition of good versus poor teaching method. Within this definition, good teaching necessarily becomes teaching which results in an actual deepening of the student's understanding of psychiatric problems, with minimum incidental damage to the patient in the process. In order to achieve such results, a teaching plan should presumably include the following: 1) selection of a student group mature enough to assimilate psychiatric material; 2) clearly defined objectives in the learning experience; 3) carefully planned supervision of the individual student; 4) systematic evaluation of results; 5) ample time in the clinic (and "ample" would require something vastly in excess of what is now allotted).

Since teaching constitutes at best an extensive investment of time on the part of both psychiatrists and students, it seems legitimate to examine the examples of psychiatric teaching above in terms of the foregoing definition of good teaching and its requisites. The first fact to be noted is that both teaching clinics under discussion are giving their teaching resources exclusively to medical students of whom only a very few will become psychiatrists. Even more significant, only one of them is investing its teaching time in the most mature medical students. One would certainly recommend that the cost of teaching facilities be weighed with all the care possible against the fact that the beneficiaries of these existing resources are in a poor position to profit adequately from the experience which is made available. This whole problem would seem to call for a fresh evaluation, partly from the point of view of when psychiatric material can most profitably be introduced in the total course of medical training, and partly from the point of view of the appropriateness of psychiatric training in clinics for medical students in contrast with the prospective psychiatrist.

The problem of clearly defining the objectives of teaching would also seem to deserve further thought. The pattern followed at Clinic B strongly suggests the underlying assumption that mere exposure to dramatic examples of psychiatric deviation is likely to prepare the average medical student for detecting and understanding psychiatric disorders in his private practice. Seemingly, the path which has been followed at Clinic C leads to more realistic results, at least it would seem that the student with experience in this clinic carries with him a greater degree of sensitivity to patients in general and a more dependable alertness to different manifestations of mental disturbance. So far as is known, there has been no real follow-up of any student group to verify the final values of psychiatry as now presented. Such follow-up commends itself in terms of simple common sense and is obviously urgently needed.

A recent appraisal of psychiatric education [5] quotes many statements indicating the doctor's dissatisfaction with the emphasis on the psychoses and urging a much greater stressing of minor psychiatric problems, the neuroses and psychosomatic conditions.

Student supervision seems an equally unexplored area

within present teaching plans. At Clinic B the emphasis appears to be placed somewhat more on a demonstration of interviewing and of patient handling which the student is encouraged to imitate or copy. At Clinic C, on the other hand, there is more opportunity for discussion between student and supervisor and perhaps in consequence, wider scope for development of the student's personal initiative.

The need for total evaluation of the teaching process in clinics is quite clear. This study was conducted quite frankly from the standpoint of benefit to the patient; and, to the extent that the patient's interests and the interests of the community colored the total approach, it is only fair to suggest that our comments on the teaching aspect of clinic work may be somewhat biased. Even allowing for this bias, it is only too apparent that a fresh view of the place of teaching within the total clinic scheme could not possibly be amiss. At the very least, it would seem desirable for each teaching clinic to answer for itself a few simple and direct questions, the responses to which should offer partial means for evaluation. One would include among these questions:

1. What are we attempting to convey in our teaching process and how do we expect it to be used? That is, what is the purpose of teaching psychiatry in this form to this group?

2. What results can we point to as the product of the teaching plan?

3. Do the results justify the present investment of psychiatric time?

4. What changes might insure better results?

5. Is it possible to do a reasonable job with the time allotted at even the best schools, or is it necessary to face realistically the absolute need for much more time to accomplish this goal?

15. PSYCHIATRIC CONSULTATION IN A GENERAL HOSPITAL

I SHOULD LIKE to discuss the subject of psychiatric consultation in a general hospital by setting forth my own personal experiences in a variety of hospitals over a period of some thirty years and to draw some conclusions from these experiences, with special emphasis on the changes which have occurred during this time.

It will be understood and, I hope, accepted that my comments about hospitals and people I have known are not so much critical as historical, since the conditions which prevailed in one were pretty much duplicated in all; we all rather grew up together, learning through trial and error and from the increasing body of knowledge about the interrelationships between personality, the emotions, and disease. What is at present called psychosomatic medicine was in its beginnings and actually reached its current, quite sophisticated development during the years of which I speak.

When I began my internship at the Beth Israel Hospital in New York in 1924 there was no psychiatrist attached to the hospital; instead there were several neuropsychiatrists whose training, skills, interests, and knowledge were all largely concerned with neurology. Except for the most manifest psychoses, which usually occurred following surgery and in the course of infectious illnesses then commonly accompanied by prolonged high fever, psychiatry was entirely ignored, if not unknown. A principal neuropsychiatrist at the hospital was a staunch devotee of the "malingerer" illusion; every patient suffering from an emotional disease was marked "suspect" in his book unless rescued by the discovery of organic changes; and the therapy was punitive, judgmental, harsh and, need I add, almost invariably unsuccessful. One goal, however, was routinely achieved: the patient would leave the hospital as quickly as possible and we would be rid of another neurotic who had been occupying precious space needed for those who were "really" sick.

Such a goal was easily accomplished by a variety of techniques: unwillingness or inability to understand, insinuation of guilt and blame and, even more devastating, accusations of willful misbehavior. Overt hostility expressed either in smirking, condescending remarks, or harsh physical procedures, and where possible, utter neglect, practically always achieved the objective; and, what is more, often led to a denial of symptoms through repression, enabling the "psychiatrist" to discharge the patient as "improved!"

To be fair about it, little indeed was known or understood in 1924 about the types of problems which then, as now, were so common on the wards of the hospital. I recall vividly the intelligent, quick, interested, and very anxious young man whose diabetes was impossible to control. This was, of course, a very serious problem in those days when the use of insulin was not universal, and the house staff was diligent in its efforts to help him. One day the mystery was solved when he was found hoisting a huge sandwich up to the ward on a rope, said sandwich supplied by his well-meaning but ignorant family. He was promptly discharged as an uncooperative patient; I wonder what would have been the reaction if someone had suggested that we inquire why a young man, fully capable of understanding the consequences of his behavior, still persisted in it. So far as I can recall, not only did no one know; no one asked and hence no answers were required.

Perhaps even more striking examples of this lack were to be found in the clinic for peripheral vascular diseases. As was to have been expected with a hospital population largely made up of Eastern European, cigarette-smoking Jews, there was a high incidence of thromboangitis obliterans. Whatever the lacks in our knowledge of the pathophysiology of this disease may have been, we knew even then that it was absolutely necessary for these patients to stop smoking. For many of them, however, no threat sufficed—no pleading, no demonstration of the catastrophic amputations certainly awaiting them if they failed to stop smoking. It was not until a good many years later that it occurred to the doctors that there must be a profound, if obscure, reason for such self-destructive behavior: an emotional problem requiring skilled psychiatric understanding and management.

Things changed materially and for the better when I got to Mount Sinai Hospital, where I was to work in one or another capacity for twenty years, although it was still a far cry from a psychiatric utopia; not only a long way from the psychiatric service which exists there and in many other general hospitals today, but also far from anything which might even by a charitable definition be called adequate. However, there were the reverberations of a beginning revolution in thinking about many problems, and there were a few inspired and dedicated psychiatrists. Their presence made a great and lasting difference.

In 1913 Clarence P. Oberndorf [1] had organized within

the Department of Neurology a psychiatric clinic, of whose existence no official notice was taken until 1924. It had then gained sufficient respectability to achieve quasi-independence even though, at that late date, it still had to hide behind the euphemistic title of "Mental Health Class." This obvious avoidance device was designed to hide the fact that the hospital was harboring within its walls a psychiatric clinic. This was, so far as I can learn, the first psychoanalytic clinic attached to a general hospital in this country.

In a paper [2] which makes most interesting and informative reading, called "The Psychiatric Clinic in a General Hospital," published in 1925, Oberndorf described the clinic at Mount Sinai Hospital. I must not pause to discuss it at length, fascinating though that would be; I should like only to emphasize a few of his major points. In the first place, he laid great emphasis on the social, community aspects of such a clinic and on the positive values of providing these services outside of the dreaded confines of the mental hospital. He also stressed the importance of the ancillary services, especially occupational therapy, social work, and recreation. He recognized the advantages to psychiatry itself of being able to draw on the medical facilities of a general hospital, mentioning in particular certain recent advances in medicine, endocrinology for example, which he felt might shed light on certain psychiatric problems. And, perhaps most important of all, he emphasized the great need to treat the medical and other patients referred to the clinic and to treat them intensively. Thus he writes, "In a few cases of conversion hysteria and compulsion neurosis, a brief psychoanalysis following the technique of Freud and devoting over a half hour three times a week to the patient has been undertaken with satisfactory results."

In those days, Oberndorf's co-workers in this clinic in-

cluded Lorand, Schonfeld, Silverberg, Broadwin, Spencer
Strauss, and Monroe Meyer. At times all these people, especially Oberndorf and Lorand, worked on the wards,
sharing an unbelievable burden of work with little or no
help.

What lay ahead can perhaps best be measured by a brief
look at hospital philosophy and the doctor-patient relationships of those days. Although I blush to recall it, I can still
remember all too well the vomitus of an hysterial patient
collected in a basin and left at his bedside with the ad-
monition that unless he stopped this nonsense, the next
time he vomited he would be refed the vomitus, by tube if
necessary. Or the heated metal rod that was inserted by
rectum if the patient did not "behave." Or the electrode
inserted in an enuretic patient's urethra.

If proof is needed of the courage and farsightedness of
Obie and his co-workers, you have it in the simple fact that
they were never deterred by the incredible hostility and
antagonism to psychiatry and psychoanalysis which existed at that time. Herman Selinsky, who began his residency at the same time as I, commented in a recent letter
about the memorial volume published in honor of Israel
Strauss, "It is wonderful to see how much psychiatry has at
long last become a legitimate and respected member of the
medical family. The youngsters are disbelieving about the
sadistic contempt and scorn which were heaped on the
heads of the previous generation."

How did this hostility manifest itself? In the first place,
despite a seeming interest and acceptance of the value of
psychiatric consultation, its use was consistently limited to
two types of patients: the utterly hopeless and the utterly
trivial. Thus, a patient with ulcerative colitis would be
"worked up" over a period of weeks, including repeated
proctoscopic examinations, x-rays, etc.; would be treated by

medications, diet and sedatives; would be watched while he slowly deteriorated; and then, finally, the psychiatrist would be invited to perform his vaunted magic. I need not emphasize the fact that no psychiatrist did indeed think he had any magical tricks up his sleeve; and certainly not in so hostile a climate, where one tip-toed gently and sometimes offered an idea or two with the deepest humility.

To be sure, we bragged a bit about our successes and, perhaps prompted by vanity and goaded by the implicit challenge to "show me," sometimes undertook the treatment of patients really beyond help from psychiatry, especially with the minimal time and the few people then available.

The trivial are more difficult to describe but equally distinct as a group. A poor suffering person would say "I wish I were dead," and the psychiatrist would be summoned posthaste to see a "suicidal" patient, often in the middle of the night. The threat should have been recognized as something less than ominous, especially when one recalls that most of these patients were Old World Jews, and that in its Yiddish form this was one of the more common laments, not too far removed from the G.I.'s "Oh, my aching back!"

Another patient might make a passing comment to an intern about some minor personal problem not even germane to the illness for which he was hospitalized; promptly an order would be left to call the psychiatrist. Often, when we finally saw him, days later, we were greeted with frank amazement by a patient who had long since forgotten the discussion which presumably occasioned the consultation in the first place.

It should be recognized, of course, that occasionally what looked like hostility was indeed merely the expression of anxiety on the part of the referring person. (Dr. Norman Reider, in commenting on this paper, said, "I saw a consultation today on a woman with a mild postoperative anxiety reaction. I prescribed Miltown: one 100 mg. tablet a day for her and three for her physician.") It is relatively easy to understand such anxiety in the novice or untrained personnel; it is not so plain why such "threats" or even the slightest expression of emotionality should create anxiety in physicians and others, often long experienced in the management of patients. Certainly, it is the psychiatric consultant's job to understand and allay such anxiety in hospital personnel since it so often results in hostility and unsympathetic handling, and ultimately in an increase of the patient's own anxieties. Thus a vicious cycle of mismanagement is set up, obviously deleterious to the best interests of the patient.

Then there were the jokes, cruel and painful. Most of them, as I remember it, were directed at two sore spots: our presumed preoccupation with sex and our failures.

Obviously, the psychiatrist's primary role is the treatment of the sick. Increasingly, he has been able to contribute to treatment in a general hospital through more accurate knowledge of psychodynamics, greater knowledge and skill in the management of emotional crises associated with organic illness, and through proper referral for psychotherapy of patients seen in consultation.

In such illnesses as asthma, hypertension, ulcerative colitis, peptic ulcer, and hyperthyroidism, the role of the emotional factors has become increasingly clear, if not as yet by any means finally and completely understood.

In the management of such crises as preoperative panics, postoperative confusional states, the pernicious vomiting of pregnancy, thyroid storms, etc., the role of the psychiatric consultant is of the first importance.

In most general hospitals the psychiatric consultant has little opportunity to undertake much treatment on the wards of the hospital. The steady demand for consultation, the lack of privacy on the wards, and the time required for individual psychotherapy make it almost impossible, except in relatively acute situations. But the consultant has an essential role to play in the screening of patients for referral to the outpatient department for therapy. Since not all patients can or should be treated, this selective process is of major importance, and is more subtle and complicated than might appear at first glance. In this there is no substitute for the clinical sense that grows out of this particular kind of experience.

The request for psychiatric consultation is a rather more complicated situation than is generally true when other specialists are asked to see hospital patients. The indications are often far less clear-cut and their significance more complex and obscure.

In the first place, and despite all our efforts at education, people generally dread "psychiatric" help and are apt to react with anxiety, resentment, or even flight to the mere suggestion that a psychiatrist be called in consultation. I am sure it is a disappointment to us all to recognize this, but it must be faced. We hear it from our medical colleagues day in and day out and experience it ourselves, especially in contacts with new patients; we still find the most archaic misinformation about psychiatrists and quite primitive attitudes even in people from whom one would not have expected such a response on the strength of their general level of education and intelligence. The fact is that the protest, "I'm not crazy; why do I need a psychiatrist?" is almost a reflex, even though it may often be expressed more subtly and indirectly.

I have already mentioned anxiety in the referring person as a possible cause for the misuse of the psychiatric referral. Another common practice is that of calling in the psychiatrist only at the point where the patient has become a problem in management and is making a nuisance of himself to the personnel or the administration ("If you don't behave yourself, I'll call the psychiatrist!"). This is easy to understand, and I would be the last one to make light of the tremendous burdens carried by these who are responsible for the care of hospitalized patients, especially in large groups on wards. But it should be emphasized that the only valid criteria for psychiatric consultation should be the nature of the patient's illness and a reasonable estimate of the potential benefit to the patient of such a consultation.

There are many other facets of psychiatric consultation, some of which warrant at least brief mention. The question of psychiatric notes on patients' charts raises special problems, both as to confidentiality and the possible use of the material in legal actions, especially if it is of a "nonmedical" (social, personal) nature. To avoid such difficulties it is now common practice to enter a brief statement noting the psychiatrist's visit, while the actual contents of the interview are recorded elsewhere and remain confidential. This device is at best a makeshift; the basic problem remains unsolved.

The simple statement of a diagnostic impression that usually results from a psychiatric consultation is less than satisfactory. Ideally, there should be an opportunity for discussion of the patient by the referring person, nurse, caseworker, and psychiatrist. This would be manifestly unrealistic in most situations, but the fact remains that many psychiatric consultations fail to contribute as much as they might to the patients' well-being and the education of hospital personnel because of this isolation from those who must carry day-to-day responsibility for treatment.

The psychiatrist himself is often handicapped by inadequate information about the patient he is to see: a brief note requesting the consultation but seldom including the reasons for the request. Many consultations lead to the recommendation that the patient be referred for treatment; unfortunately, the psychiatrist seldom learns of the outcome of his prescription. Whether the psychiatrist should assume more responsibility for following up on the patient's progress or the referring person should keep the psychiatrist informed of developments is not the issue. The crucial problem here is a breakdown in communication which can only result in less than optimal service to patients and a generally frustrating and unrewarding experience for the staff.

After all my years of work in general hospitals I believe that the psychiatrist's greatest contribution has been and in a sense still is the growing recognition of the worth of the individual patient, of the dignity and value of the human spirit, and the necessity for considering the patient as a feeling person. This may seem naïve and unscientific, but it is my conviction.

The dehumanized attitude toward the patient which had become quite prevalent in medicine in the guise of science and had been catalyzed by enormous strides in pathology, physiology, endocrinology, etc., was relatively new in the 1920s, as new as the budding specialty of psychoanalysis. Much earlier, the physician had this regard for the whole human, the person, which was handed down naturally and inevitably by his priestly forebears. For a long time the general practitioner, the almost legendary family doctor, had occupied an analogous role, only to give way in an age of scientific medicine to specialization and the array of scientific tools. As Alexander [3] pointed out:

Disease meant now no longer what happens to the whole man but what happens to his organs. . . . And so the natural and original mission of the physician, the approach to disease as a whole changes into the small task of localising the ailment and identifying it and ascribing it to an already specific group of diseases. . . . This unavoidable objectification and technicalization of therapy in the 19th century came to an extreme excess because between the physician and the patient became interpolated a third entirely mechanical thing, the apparatus. The penetrating, creative synthesizing grasp of the born physician became less and less necessary for diagnosis.

And Alan Gregg: [4]

The totality that is a human being has been divided for study into parts and systems; one cannot decry the method but one is not obliged to remain satisfied with its results alone. What brings and keeps our several organs and numerous functions in harmony and federation? And what has medicine to say of the facile separation of "mind" and "body?" What makes an individual what the word implies—not divided? The need for more knowledge here is of an excruciating obviousness. But more than mere need there is a foreshadowing of changes to come. Psychiatry is astir, neurophysiology is crescent, neurosurgery flourishes, and a star still hangs over the cradle of endocrinology. . . . Contributions from other fields are to seek from psychology, cultural anthropology, sociology, and philosophy as well as from chemistry and physics and internal medicine to resolve the dichotomy of mind and body left us by Descartes.

It was really the emphasis on the whole man that ultimately helped change the attitude of the physician, and especially the psychoanalytic awareness of the meaningfulness of all the patient's symptoms no matter how difficult this might be to accept at first glance. We have obviously made real progress toward this goal.

Gradually the psychiatrist appearing on the wards is coaxing the doctor out from behind his white coat and dangling stethoscope to take a look at a man and to talk with him and, most of all perhaps, to be willing to listen and try to understand.

I have told this incident to a generation of students and residents but I hope it will bear still another telling. Patients with hyperthyroidism were treated at Mount Sinai Hospital in the 1920s by a method devised by Kessel and Hyman [5] which they called, euphemistically, "skillful neglect." Despite their awareness that emotional factors were involved, at least in precipitating the illness, the treatment consisted essentially of bed rest, warm packs, sedation, and frequent feedings of food with high caloric value. It also consisted, obviously and importantly, of making the patient feel "special," one of a favored few, the object of special concern on the part of the nurses, house staff, and particularly the "chief," the professor, if you will. I need not elaborate the psychological factors involved in the apparent success of such treatment in gratifying every infantile wish, oral, tactile, narcissistic, etc.

One day a patient with hyperthyroidism was admitted to the Neurological Service for reasons that had nothing to do with the patient or her illness. At any rate she came under the management of the neurologist, and Obie sort of bootlegged me into being her psychiatrist. It was then early in my residency in neurology, and my psychiatric education had been limited indeed. [6] I had never even taken a psychiatric history. When I begged Obie to tell me what to do, he suggested that I talk to the patient about herself and listen carefully to anything she had to say. This I did and gradually a person unfolded—hopes, illusions, disappointments, crises, conflicts, defenses, and all—and with Obie's gentle prodding and some very hard work, I gained my first awareness of an entirely new dimension in the relationship of doctor and patient.

This may seem quite trivial, but it is just this shift in emphasis, in values, in tolerance and understanding, that I think is so fundamental. No longer is the doctor limited to

the study of an ill-functioning or diseased organ; no longer
need he be exclusively concerned with the mass, the speci-
men, the chemical calculation, the changes in electrical con-
ductivity. No longer need the main object of study and
concern be this "interesting" mass to be palpated or that
"wonderful" sound on the inside to be picked up, all subsequently to be discussed within the hearing if not the
comprehension of the patient.

One of the first things I learned from Obie and others was
respect for the sick person. This went beyond sympathy
and patience and beyond devoted attention to the illness, all
of which were deeply imbedded in the philosophy of the
hospital. Respect included a different dimension of understanding the worth of the person and the meaning to him of
his sickness and all the experiences associated with his
treatment.

Talking to a group of general practitioners ten years ago,
Rennie recalled that when he was an intern they went on
"grand rounds" and wheeled about large cases of autopsy
material—kidneys, lungs, or some other pathological sub-
stances illustrating what the patient was presumably suffering from: [7]

We wheeled these out before the patient, and we discussed
in front of him all the details of his condition in a conversation
which might go somewhat like one I heard a week ago in a
large hospital in New York City. A seventeen-year-old boy
lay in his bed, and about twenty doctors were grouped around
him. They discussed the pros and cons of what the pathology
in his abdomen might be. One doctor said, "I think he has a
hypernephroma." Another offered his tentative diagnosis, and
a third said, "Why he's exactly like that patient we had on the
third floor a couple of months ago." Someone asked, "What
happened to him?" "Oh, he died. He died last week." A fifth
doctor said, "Have we any slides of this thing?" Whereupon

another doctor said, "Of course we haven't any slides; the patient is still living." Then the doctor who had asked about the slides said, "Well, we'll probably get them in a couple of months from now." And the seventeen-year-old patient lay in bed listening to this conversation.

This attitude toward the patients, especially as seen on rounds, was one of the most disturbing things to me. Not only did it seem that no thought was given to how such rounds might be used positively in the management of the patients; they were often highly destructive and, paradoxically, the perpetrators were essentially kind and devoted men.

It is my impression that the presence of the psychiatrist and his active participation, both as consultant and member of the team on a given service, medical or surgical, have made for considerable improvement in the management of rounds, especially in the avoidance of the shocking and demoralizing bedside discussions of the patient. However, a recently published and highly illuminating study by Kaufman, Franzblau, and Kairys [8] at Mount Sinai Hospital suggests that the wish may be, at least in part, responsible for this impression. Although the study had a much wider scope than this particular aspect of hospital care, some of the reported incidents, such as the discussion of a patient's terminal illness in her presence, indeed seem to turn back the clock.

The psychiatrist can do much to implement this study's emphasis on "the need for respect for the patient's person and privacy," which is indeed a major premise of psychiatry itself. The psychiatrist knows and can teach his colleagues such things as the meaning of the authoritarian role played by the "big doctor, the chief"; can demonstrate that even the patient who seems most withdrawn and too sick to understand, does hear and must ruminate on the meaning of the half-understood and barely perceived comment; and can try to make clear to his colleagues the influence of all such emotional stresses on a patient's illness and recovery.

One of the inevitable by-products of this new interest in the patient as a person is the increased readiness of the hospital staff to observe and respond to deviations in the patient's behavior. This is true for doctors—especially the interns and residents—nurses, social workers, and occupational therapists, among others. Although he is generally asked to see a patient, as consultant, by the physician in charge, it is not at all rare these days for a nurse who has observed some bizarre piece of behavior in a patient or been made party to some anxiety-producing confidence to ask through the appropriate channels that a psychiatrist be called in consultation.

More importantly, a growing bond of usefulness and skill collaboration has developed between the social service and psychiatric departments as they have, in a sense, grown up together. Although this is not the place to discuss it, the interaction between the social emphasis of casework and the dynamic (psychoanalytic) insights of psychiatry has many fascinating and significant ramifications. Suffice it to say here that each has contributed to the other, formally and informally. Today social work has its own highly developed therapeutic armamentarium in which, when indicated, it may judiciously use psychiatric consultation. Similarly, psychiatry has learned to make effective use of the skills of casework in what has become, in and out of the traditional clinical team approach, a most fruitful and happy collaboration.

The psychiatrist teaches as he goes, literally as well as figuratively. Of all the teaching tools I know, none is more effective than discussion by the psychiatric consultant of a patient or group of patients on the ward or in a clinic with those directly responsible for the actual care of patients. I have never ceased to delight in the interchange among nurse, social worker, resident, and psychiatrist in the informal atmosphere of the day room, and its educational potential. Of course, I do not mean to imply that the tremendous advances in these professions have resulted from such informal infiltration of psychiatric ideas alone, but they have helped, I think, more than is generally recognized.

One of the chief beneficiaries of the educational role inherent in psychiatric consultation in a general hospital has been the psychiatrist himself. When the psychiatrist emerged from the psychiatric hospital where his work had been restricted to the care of the mentally ill, and began to work actively with this group of general medical and surgical patients, he added a whole new dimension to his work and an opportunity for a type of experience he had previously been denied. This taught him a very different approach to illness and afforded new and startling illustrations of his developing psychodynamic formulations. Out of this, indeed, grew a whole new branch of psychiatric practice, psychosomatic medicine. Indeed, as we are only now beginning to realize, we went too far in this quasi-specialization, and corrective insights are already being applied.

Most of all, psychiatry can give the doctor the tools to understand the person and to learn the meaning of the symptoms and the illness. No doctor thus armed can ever again neglect the patient in his human aspects or slight the dignity of his human needs and wants. "In their simplest form the ingredients of dynamic understanding and relationship can be reduced to the words respect and affection. If you like an individual for himself, you can disapprove of something he does while continuing to like him; if you respect him as a human being, you assume his right to think

and feel as he does and to be the kind of person he is." [9]
Assuming this, the doctor who wishes to treat a patient must
try to understand how and why he thinks and feels as he
does, insofar as his feelings affect and are in turn affected
by the illness which brings him to the doctor. I would only
like to repeat that I believe this may in the end prove to
have been the psychiatrist's greatest contribution to medical
care in the general hospital.

NOTES

1. MENTAL HEALTH: THEORETICAL ASSUMPTIONS

1. Clifford Beers, *A Mind That Found Itself* (New York, Doubleday & Co., 1950, revised ed.). First published 1908.

2. In 1950 the National Committee for Mental Hygiene joined with the National Mental Health Foundation and the Psychiatric Foundation to form the National Association for Mental Health. This shift in title represents something more than a merely administrative device. In general there is now a tendency to use the term "mental health" rather than "mental hygiene" in such organizational titles and elsewhere.

3. Letter to Beers, *A Mind That Found Itself*, p. 265.

4. It is interesting to note that in his first letter concerning a new society for mental hygiene, Meyer said that "something must be done to meet one of the most difficult but also lamentably neglected problems of *sociological* improvement" (my italics), thus at the outset recognizing factors beyond the clinical or strictly psychiatric. In Beers, *A Mind That Found Itself*, p. 264.

5. I. S. Wechsler, "The Legend of the Prevention of Mental Disease," *Journal of the American Medical Association*, XCV (1930), 24.

6. Herbert S. Jennings, John B. Watson, Adolf Meyer, and William I. Thomas, *Suggestions of Modern Science Concerning Education* (New York, Macmillan Co., 1925), p. 118.

7. Sol W. Ginsburg, "Values and the Psychiatrist," *American Journal of Orthopsychiatry*, XX (1950), 468.

8. Kingsley Davis, "Mental Hygiene and the Class Structure," *Psychiatry*, I (1938), 55.

9. For a full documentation of this comment, see Robert Tyson, "Current Mental Hygiene Practice," *Journal of Clinical Psychology*, Vol. VII, No. 1, Monograph Supplement 1951.

10. M. J. Rosenau, "Mental Hygiene and Public Health," *Mental Hygiene*, XIX (1935), 9.

11. Walter Bromberg, *The Mind of Man* (New York, Harper & Brothers, 1937), p. 217.

12. Tyson, "Current Mental Hygiene Practice," *Journal of Clinical Psychology*, Vol. VII, No. 1, Monograph Supplement 1951.

13. Davis, "Mental Hygiene and the Class Structure," *Psychiatry*, I (1938), 55.

14. A more detailed, more carefully considered "working" definition is given in the pamphlet entitled *Mental Health Is: 1, 2, 3* (New York, National Association for Mental Health, 1951).

15. Wechsler, "The Legend of the Prevention of Mental Disease," *Journal of the American Medical Association*, XCV (1930), 24.

16. Robert Knight, "Plans for the Study of the Epidemiology of Mental Disorder: Most Urgent Problems to Be Investigated," in *Epidemiology of Mental Disorder* (New York, Milbank Memorial Fund, 1950).

17. Erich Lindemann, in *Epidemiology of Mental Disorder*, p. 34.

18. Yet it is saddening to realize that at this late date, in a survey in a large city (St. Louis), only about one third of the sample tested knew that hospital conditions were poor. M. Tabackman, "Knowledge and Opinion of Mental Health," *Smith College Studies in Social Work*, XXI, No. 3 (1951), 261.

19. George S. Stevenson, "The Mental Health Program in Perspective," *Mental Hygiene*, XXXV, No. 1 (1951), 5 ff.

20. Frankwood E. Williams, "Development of Mental Hygiene," in Sandor Lorand, ed., *Psychoanalysis Today: Its Scope and Function* (New York, Covici, Friede, 1933).

21. Nina Ridenour, "Mental Hygiene Education," in *Orthopsychiatry 1923–1948: Retrospect and Prospect* (New York, American Orthopsychiatric Association, 1948), p. 566.

22. Important research on attitude change is in progress at various universities; the results should be of the greatest value to mental hygiene.

23. See, in this connection, Kurt Lewin and Paul Grabbe, "Conduct, Knowledge and Acceptance of New Values," *Journal of Social Issues*, I (1945), 53–63.

24. Gregory Zilboorg, "The Mental Health Aspect of the Communication of Ideas," in F. R. Moulton and P. O. Komora, eds., *Mental Health*, publication of the American Association for the Advancement of Science, No. 9 (Lancaster, Pa., The Science Press, 1939), p. 283.

25. See Jeanne Watson, "Some Social and Psychological Situations Related to Change in Attitude," *Human Relations*, III (1950), 15. In this illuminating and relevant study, Watson discusses four stages in the process of attitude change which I believe bear out this analogy: (1) a predisposition to change; (2) a more or less generalized change in which (3) attention is directed to the inadequacy of the particular attitude and it is changed accordingly; and (4) reinforcement of the new attitude. She concludes that "change in attitude must also mean change in related social attitudes and personality structure." It may be fairly said that these conditions exist in the educational situations in which immersion in mental hygiene principles seems most successful. This is well known but apparently not always kept in mind in planning educational activities. It seems to be an absolutely basic principle.

26. Ernst Kris, "On Psychoanalysis and Education," *American Journal of Orthopsychiatry*, XVIII (1948), 623.

27. An exception to this is to be found in the usual college textbooks on what is euphemistically called "mental hygiene." An examination of a number of these (there are a great many) reveals a curious combination of clinical psychiatry, abnormal psychology, undemonstrated "facts" about personality, and good, old-fashioned advice, not excluding simple error. Thus, in one of these texts one reads, in a discussion of schizophrenia: "The [schizophrenic] may become rigid and stubborn, his eyes [sic] may dilate and his body may quiver if he is forced to do something against his will." Or again, in a discussion of personality types: "In this development of the psychoanalytic theory of personality types, Freud and his followers appear to stress the effect upon personality of environmentally stimulated satisfactions and frustrations as related to psycho-sexual development. These types represent abnormal rather than normal adjustment." Or, in a discussion of blind dates: "Pickup boys and girls are social misfits and engage in the behavior solely for self-satisfaction."

28. For a fuller and characteristically incisive discussion of this question, see Kris, "On Psychoanalysis and Education," *American Journal of Orthopsychiatry*, XVIII (1948).

29. Willie Hoffer, "Psychoanalytic Education," in *The Psychoanalytic Study of the Child* (New York, International Universities Press, 1945), I, 299.

30. See *Promotion of Mental Health in the Primary and Secondary Schools: An Evaluation of Four Projects*, Group for the Advancement of Psychiatry, Report No. 18, Jan., 1951.

31. Certain of these training programs have yielded valuable insights into the educational and emotional aspects of this kind of group learning process. This process is considered in the reports of two institutes, one for general practitioners and the other for public health workers, both held under the aegis of The Commonwealth Fund: (1) Helen L. Witmer, ed., *Teaching Psychotherapeutic Medicine: An Experimental Course for General Physicians* (New York, The Commonwealth Fund, 1947); (2) Ethel L. Ginsburg, *Public Health Is People: An Institute on Mental Health in Public Health* (New York, The

Commonwealth Fund, 1950). Both books are now published by Harvard University Press, Cambridge, Mass.

32. Lawrence K. Frank, "Social Order and Psychiatry," *American Journal of Ortho-psychiatry*, XI (1941), 620 ff.

33. Samuel Whitman, "Organizing for Mental Health in the Local Community," in *Social Work in the Current Scene* (New York, Columbia University Press, 1950).

34. Kris, "On Psychoanalysis and Education," *American Journal of Orthopsychiatry*, XVIII (1948).

35. H. V. Dicks, "In Search of Our Proper Ethic," *British Journal of Medical Psychology*, XXIII (1950), 1.

36. H. V. Dicks, "Principles of Mental Hygiene," in Noel G. Harris, ed., *Modern Trends in Psychological Medicine* (London, Butterworth & Co., 1948), pp. 310 ff.

37. It is worth noting that in Dicks' concept of mental hygiene "treatment" and "prevention" are intermingled.

38. Marie Jahoda, *Methodological Problems in the Psychoanalytic Approach to the Study of Social Issues.* Read at the meeting of the American Psychoanalytic Association, Washington, D.C., May 15, 1948.

39. Whether or not one agrees with the nuances of Dicks' psychoanalytic formulations (as, for instance, his designation of a "strong social stereotype of respectability and status aspiration" as "an anal-erotic behavior pattern"), the value of his mental hygiene theory, as of any other, has to be tested by how it may be utilized prophylactically.

40. See also, e.g., *The Mental Hygiene Bulletin* published by the Michigan Mental Hygiene Society, VIII (1950), No. 4.

41. See Marie Jahoda, "Emotional Predispositions to Prejudice," *Intercultural Education News*, IX (1948), Nos. 3–4, p. 6: "It is conceded that prejudice is a social phenomenon, not an invention of the neurotic mind, and should be subjected to interdisciplinary investigation. The psychiatric approach nevertheless seems to offer the possibility of essential insights which could not be discovered by other disciplines."

42. See, in this connection, Ethel L. Ginsburg, *Public Health Is People*, pp. 17, 171, 234.

2. THE NEUROSES

1. In this connection see Marie Jahoda, *Toward a Social Psychology of Mental Health; in Problems of Infancy and Childhood* (New York, Josiah H. Macy, Jr. Foundation, 1950), and the leaflet *Mental Health Is: 1, 2, 3* (New York, National Association for Mental Health, 1951). For a definition from the psychoanalytic point of view, see L. S. Kubie, *Practical and Theoretical Aspects of Psychoanalysis* (New York, International Universities Press, 1950), pp. 13–14.

2. By "clinically significant" is meant of an order of severity and consequence to justify seeking and obtaining appropriate medical or other assistance. Occasionally others who associate with a person (family, employer, fellow workers) may be aware of the need for help before the individual himself can recognize or acknowledge that such need exists.

3. See, for definitive data, Eli Ginzberg and Associates, *The Ineffective Soldier*, Volume I: *The Lost Divisions* (New York, Columbia University Press, 1959), *passim*.

4. E. A. Strecker, "Psychiatric Education," *Mental Hygiene*, XIV (1930), 797.

5. F. C. McLean, "Psychiatry and General Medicine," *Mental Hygiene*, XVI (1932), 577.

6. P. H. Salmond, "Importance and Value of the Psychiatric Ward in Public and Private General Hospitals," *Diseases of the Nervous System*, V (1944), 233.

7. National Association for Mental Health, *Facts and Figures about Mental Illness* (New York, The Association, 1952), p. 14.

8. Statement by Dr. Martha Eliot, chief of the Children's Bureau, at a meeting on juvenile delinquency called by the National Social Welfare Assembly, July, 1952.

9. National Association for Mental Health, *Facts and Figures about Mental Illness*, p. 14.

10. F. Alexander, *Fundamentals of Psychoanalysis* (New York, W. W. Norton & Co., 1948), pp. 199–200.

11. The terms "ego" and "superego" are used in their Freudian sense. The ego represents the conscious, rational aspects of the personality; it makes inner and outer experiences conscious, controls movements and actions, and mediates between the demands of the instincts, of the superego, and of reality. The superego represents the conscience, that is, the internalized commands of parents and other authorities and the ideals of the personality. In this latter function it is sometimes called the ego-ideal.

12. A defense mechanism is used by the personality whenever the ego is threatened and fails in its integrative function. Such defenses include rationalization, projection, repression, and many others. These defenses are sometimes used by normal people in commonplace life situations; they are, however, much more often encountered in neurotics and psychotics. For a fuller discussion, see Alexander, *Fundamentals of Psychoanalysis*, Chap. V, pp. 82–138.

13. *Ibid.*, pp. 214–15.

14. In Freudian terms such impulses are considered as part of the id, which represents the unconscious drives and all the instincts of the personality.

15. I. S. Wechsler, *The Neurologist's Point of View* (New York, L. B. Fischer Publishing Corp., 1945), p. 251.

16. R. P. Knight, "An Evaluation of Psychotherapeutic Techniques," *Bulletin of the Menninger Clinic*, XVI, No. 4 (1952), 113.

17. Kubie, *Practical and Theoretical Aspects of Psychoanalysis*, p. 21.

18. Knight, "An Evaluation of Psychotherapeutic Techniques," *Bulletin of the Menninger Clinic*, XVI, No. 4 (1952), 115.

19. Kubie, *Practical and Theoretical Aspects of Psychoanalysis*, p. 1.

3. ADJUSTMENT: ITS USES AND DANGERS

1. Jahoda, *Toward a Social Psychology of Mental Health; in Problems of Infancy and Childhood.*
2. Eric Hoffer, *The True Believer* (New York, Harper & Brothers, 1951).
3. Felix Cohen, *The Reconstruction of Hidden Value Judgments in Symbols and Values* (New York, Harper & Brothers, 1954).
4. Gilbert Highet, *The Art of Teaching* (New York, Alfred A. Knopf, Inc., 1954).
5. "U.S. Kids Are O.K.," *This Week*, Feb. 27, 1955.
6. Learned Hand, *The Spirit of Liberty* (New York, Alfred A. Knopf, Inc., 1952).

5. VALUES AND THE PSYCHIATRIST

1. Micah 6:6–8.
2. Robin Williams, in *Bulletin of the American Psychoanalytic Association*, V (Sept., 1949), 41.
3. Sommers, in *Bulletin of the American Psychoanalytic Association*, V (Sept., 1949), 39.
4. John Carl Flügel, *Man, Morals and Society; a Psychoanalytical Study* (New York, International Universities Press, 1945), p. 16.
5. Erich Fromm, *Escape from Freedom* (New York, Farrar & Rinehart, Inc., 1941) and *Man for Himself; an Inquiry into the Psychology of Ethics* (New York, Rinehart & Co., Inc., 1947).
6. Eli Ginzberg and others, *Occupational Choice: An Approach to a General Theory* (New York, Columbia University Press, 1951).
7. Sigmund Freud, *An Autobiographical Study* (London, Hogarth Press, 1948), p. 26.
8. Kubie, *Practical and Theoretical Aspects of Psychoanalysis*, p. 138.

9. Sachs, "Observations of a Training Analyst," *Psychoanalytic Quarterly*, XVI (1947), 157.

10. It is interesting to recall in this connection that Freud attributed Rank's experimentation with short analysis to an attempt to keep pace with "American prosperity," suggesting that this is hardly a "recent" problem.

11. A recent report from a colleague ends with the statement: "I do not mean to accuse the patient of homosexuality. . . ." A colleague writes: "He is an immensely gifted and socially useful young writer and I hope you can take him on. . . ." etc., etc.

12. Morris Raphael Cohen, *Reason and Nature* (New York, Harcourt, Brace & Co., 1931), p. 348.

13. Gunnar Myrdal, *An American Dilemma* (New York, Harper & Brothers, 1944), Appendix 2: "A Methodological Note on Facts and Valuations in Social Science," p. 1042, gives a brilliant and invaluable statement on the entire problem, which is required reading for anyone interested in the question of values.

14. *Ibid.*, pp. 1063–64.

15. Morgenau, "Ethical Science," *Scientific Monthly*, XLIX (Nov., 1939), 290.

16. Sol W. Ginsburg, "Social Science and Social Action," *Mental Hygiene*, XXXIII, No. 2 (1949), 236.

17. Hadley Cantril, *Understanding Man's Social Behavior* (Princeton, N.J., Office of Public Opinion Research, 1948), pp. 40–41, emphasizes: "There is no fundamental difference in the *process* of value judgment or interpretation between the physical scientist and the social scientist, whether they deal with atoms, nerve conduction or everyday social behavior." "The difference between them," he continues, "is merely a difference in the complexity of the value-judgment process required in reaching higher order abstractions or 'explanations.' " Similarly, he points out, "Social scientists are frequently criticized for a lack of objectivity. But any scientist— no matter how 'pure' his research—must make value judgments as to the probable meaning of the facts he knows or uncovers

if he is to be more than a mere recorder of information. The value judgments (interpretations) the social scientist must make are complicated by the nature of the material he studies —whether in the laboratory, the survey field, the group, or via men's institutions. These purposes of others are frequently potential influences on the purposes of the social scientist himself, who is also a human being."

18. Bertrand Russell, *Authority and the Individual* (New York, Simon and Schuster, Inc., 1949).

19. In the following discussion I have relied largely on the statement of the Committee on Social Issues of the Group for the Advancement of Psychiatry, "The Social Responsibility of Psychiatry: A Statement of Orientation," and have quoted from it freely. I would urge a reading of this statement, to which my condensation scarcely does justice.

20. Another aspect of danger in the social environment is what is spoken of as the "overprotective" situation. "There are two kinds of overprotective environments. First, overprotection reflected in actual overindulgence of the individual. If this takes place in the crucial phases of personality maturation, it may weaken the personality, discourage growth, and reinforce psychopathic conduct. Second, the other type of overprotective environment is the neurotic variety, in which the alleged symbols of security and protection are false and represent actually a hostile rejection. In such instances, the overprotection is simply a guise for the denial of hate."

21. Ignazio Silone, in Richard Crossman, ed., *The God That Failed* (New York, Harper & Brothers, 1949), p. 114.

6. RELIGION AND PSYCHIATRY

1. I wish to acknowledge my indebtedness to various books from which I have derived considerable help: Gregory Zilboorg, *Mind, Medicine and Man* (New York, Harcourt, Brace & Co., 1943); Melville J. Herskovits, *Man and His Works* (New York, Alfred A. Knopf, Inc., 1948); and George Headley, *The Superstitions of the Irreligious* (New York, Macmil-

lan Co., 1951). I am sure a good percentage of my readers will count themselves among the irreligious; I would commend to them a careful reading of Headley's charming and sensitive book.

2. I am not, of course, arguing here the case for or against the belief in miracles. Not that I believe it irrelevant or sacrosanct; merely that this is obviously not the place to enter into such a discussion.

7. CULTURAL FACTORS IN SOCIAL WORK

1. One gets some notion of this from the fact, for instance, that any current issue of *Psychological Abstracts* contains references to 30–40 articles and books on this subject, not a few of which relate particularly to matters of direct concern to social workers.

2. E. B. Taylor, *Primitive Culture* (New York, 1874), p. 1.

3. Herskovits, *Man and His Works*, pp. 17 ff.

4. *Ibid.*, p. 25.

5. Sol W. Ginsburg, "Values and the Psychiatrist," *American Journal of Orthopsychiatry*, XX, No. 3 (1950).

6. There are a few exceptions to this but for our purposes it is not essential to enumerate them.

7. Herskovits, *Man and His Works*, p. 29.

8. This whole differentiation is brilliantly argued in Herskovits' book.

9. See, for instance, Solly Zuckermann, *The Social Life of Monkeys and Apes* (New York, Harcourt, Brace & Co., 1932).

10. For some interesting sidelights on this general subject, see Lyman Bryson and others, eds., *Symbols and Values: An Initial Study* (New York, Harper & Brothers, 1954).

11. Herskovits, *Man and His Works*, p. 628.

12. Margaret Mead and Rhoda B. Métraux, eds., *The Study of Culture at a Distance* (Chicago, University of Chicago Press, 1953). This volume contains an excellent bibliography.

13. *Ibid.*, p. 33.

14. Herskovits, *Man and His Works*, p. 640.

15. For some recent interesting and relevant statements on interviewing, see "The Interview as Evaluative Technique," in *Institutional Conference on Testing Problems 1953* (Princeton, N.J., Educational Testing Service, 1953). See also Merton M. Gill and others, *The Initial Interview in Psychiatric Practice* (New York, International Universities Press, 1954).

16. In this connection it is interesting that the woman to whose home they were sent by the Travelers Aid Society commented that they were both quiet, refined girls, "Indian enough not to talk too much about their private affairs."

17. Sol W. Ginsburg, *Concerning Religious Values; a Psychiatrist's Viewpoint* (Cincinnati, Ohio, Hebrew Union College, 1949).

18. The problem of chaperonage is a constant one in my dealings with adolescent children of foreign parentage. No youngster brought up on the American scene can be expected to accept gracefully, if at all, the European, Latin-American concept of chaperonage. The American dating system, that invaluable testing ground for adulthood, especially adult sexual roles, is irreconcilable with the European notion of chaperonage. Unfortunately, many parents of European birth find it impossible to accept this, probably because of conflicts of their own which they project into the situation and rationalize in cultural terms.

19. See, for instance, Sol W. Ginsburg, "The Impact of the Social Worker's Cultural Structure on Social Therapy," *Social Casework*, XXXII (Oct., 1951), 319; W. Gioseffi, "The Relationship of Culture to the Principles of Casework," *Social Casework*, XXXII (May, 1951), 190; D. Lee, "Some Implications of Culture for Interpersonal Relations," *Social Casework*, XXI (Oct., 1950), 355; P. I. Sandi, "The Psychocultural Approach in Social Casework," *Social Casework*, XXVIII, No. 10 (1947), 377; N. H. Handley, "Social Casework and Intercultural Problems," *Social Casework*, XXVIII, No. 2 (1947), 43.

20. Sol W. Ginsburg, "The Impact of the Social Worker's

Cultural Structure on Social Therapy," *Social Casework*, XXXII (Oct., 1951), 319.

21. Luna B. Brown, "Race as a Factor in Establishing Case-work Relationship," *Social Casework*, XXXI, No. 3 (1950), 91. See also I. B. Lindsay, "Race as a Factor in the Caseworker's Role," *Social Casework*, XXVIII, No. 3 (1947), 101; E. Layne, "Experience of a Negro Psychiatric Social Worker in a Veterans Administration Mental Hygiene Clinic," *Journal of Psychiatric Social Work*, XIX (1949), No. 2.

22. A recent paper indeed proposes that a patient is best treated by a member of his own race or religion. See Clarence P. Oberndorf, "Selectivity and Option for Psychiatry," *American Journal of Psychiatry*, CX, No. 8 (April, 1954), 754.

23. N. W. Ackerman and Marie Jahoda, *Anti-Semitism and Emotional Disorder* (New York, Harper & Brothers, 1950). These authors make a distinction between prejudice, pre-judgment, and stereotyping which I have not tried to follow in this discussion. The reader is referred to their text for the elaboration of their point of view.

24. Gertrud M. Kurth, "The Jew and Adolf Hitler," *The Psychoanalytic Quarterly*, XVI (1947). See also Gertrud M. Kurth, "Politics: Unconscious Factors in Social Prejudice and Mass Movements," in Hans Herma and Gertrud M. Kurth, eds., *Elements of Psychoanalysis* (New York, World Publishing Co., 1951).

25. O. Fenichel, "Elements of a Psychoanalytic Theory of Anti-Semitism," in E. Simmel, ed., *Anti-Semitism, a Social Disease* (New York, International Universities Press, 1946).

26. Max Horkheimer and Samuel H. Flowerman, eds., *Studies in Prejudice*; T. W. Adorno, Else Frenkel-Brunswik, Daniel J. Levinson, and R. Nevitt Sanford, *The Authoritarian Personality*; Bruno Bettelheim and Morris Janowitz, *Dynamics of Prejudice*; N. W. Ackerman and Marie Jahoda, *Anti-Semitism and Emotional Disorder*; Paul W. Massin, *Rehearsal for Destruction*. See also G. W. Allport, *The Nature*

of Prejudice (Cambridge, Mass., Addison Wesley Publishing Co., 1954).

27. Else Frenkel-Brunswik and R. Nevitt Sanford, "The Anti-Semitic Personality: A Research Report," in E. Simmel, ed., *Anti-Semitism, a Social Disease.*

28. Although these remarks are made about anti-Semitism, most of them will apply equally well to other analagous forms of prejudice.

29. Ackerman and Jahoda, *Anti-Semitism and Emotional Disorder*, p. 26.

30. *Ibid.*, p. 28.

31. *Ibid.*, p. 29.

32. *Ibid.*, p. 55.

33. G. Murphy, *In the Minds of Men* (New York, Basic Books, Inc., 1953).

34. Incidentally, the test for the normalcy of an attitude rests first on its reversibility when exposed to the facts!

35. Murphy, *In the Minds of Men*, pp. 222 ff.

36. See the American Jewish Committee series. See also A. Kardiner and L. Ovesey, *The Mask of Oppression: A Psychosocial Study of the American Negro* (New York, W. W. Norton & Co., 1951).

37. The problem of cultural relativity is of considerable interest and importance and deserves much fuller consideration than we can undertake here. Cultural relativity, stated in its simplest terms, "asserts that any set of customs and institutions or way of life is as valid as any other." Frank E. Hartung, "Cultural Relativity and Moral Judgments," *Philosophy of Science*, XXI, No. 2 (April, 1954), 118. The matter is hardly as simple as this, touching as it does on many basic philosophic questions, such as the problem of values, moral standards, and the ultimate nature of reality. The interested reader will find an excellent, brief discussion of this question in Herskovits, *Man and His Works*, and also in A. L. Kroeber and C. Kluckhohn, *A Critical Review of Concepts and Orientations* (Cambridge, Mass., Peabody Museum, 1952).

8. WHAT UNEMPLOYMENT DOES TO PEOPLE

1. This study was one part of a larger investigation on economics and group behavior. The staff was headed by Dr. Eli Ginzberg, economist on the staff of Columbia University, and included Mrs. Ethel L. Ginsburg, Miss Dorothy L. Lynn, Miss Mildred Vickers, and myself. A complete report of this investigation was published by Harper & Brothers under the title *The Unemployed*.

2. I have attempted in this presentation to avoid speculations not warranted by the nature and scope of the material. I believe it is by just such speculations that harm is done to the attempts at collaboration between psychiatrist and social scientist.

3. In this connection see Schmideberg, "Zum Verständnis massenpsychologischer Erscheinungen," *Imago*, XXI, 445.

4. Hans W. Singer, *Unemployment and the Unemployed* (Brooklyn, N.Y., Chemical Publishing Co., 1940).

9. THE ROLE OF WORK

1. Ernest Jones, "The Significance of Sublimating Processes in Education and Re-education," in *Papers on Psychoanalysis* (London, Bailliere, Tindal & Cox, 1923).

2. Helene Deutsch, "Some Psychoanalytic Observations in Surgery," *Psychosomatic Medicine*, IV (1942).

3. Eli Ginzberg and others, *Occupational Choice: An Approach to a General Theory* (New York, Columbia University Press, 1951).

4. Erik H. Erikson, *Childhood and Society* (New York, W. W. Norton & Co., 1950).

5. Anna Freud, *Ego and the Mechanisms of Defence.*

6. Henry H. Hart, "Workers Integration," *Medical Record*, Dec., 1947.

7. Sigmund Freud, *Civilization and Its Discontents.*

8. "An adult who is deprived of his work, his profession,

loses the essential connection of being an adult. He is made dependent on others once again, as he was in early childhood." B. Lantos, "Work and the Instincts," *International Journal of Psychiatry*, XIV (1943).

9. Eli Ginzberg and associates, *The Unemployed* (New York, Harper & Brothers, 1943).

10. WORK AND ITS SATISFACTIONS

1. I am indebted to Dr. Ginzberg for many of the insights reflected in this paper as in my other writings on this subject.

2. Eli Ginzberg and others, *The Unemployed*.

3. Sigmund Freud, *The Ego and the Id* (London, Hogarth Press, 1927).

4. Hans W. Singer, *Unemployment and the Unemployed*.

5. Erikson, *Childhood and Society*. Perhaps this notion of work as a "curse" is analagous to the use of this word as a euphemism for the menstrual period, i.e., as something not actually so bad at all, but inescapable and a continuing reminder of the woman's presumedly inferior role as an individual and in society.

6. M. E. Spiro, *Kibbutz, Venture in Utopia* (Cambridge, Mass., Harvard University Press, 1956). See also M. Weingarten, *Life in a Kibbutz* (New York, Reconstructionist Press, 1955).

7. Eli Ginzberg and others, *Occupational Choice*.

8. For a detailed discussion of these terms and of our position concerning work satisfaction, see Eli Ginzberg and others, *Occupational Choice*, especially Chapters 14 and 15.

9. Freud, *The Ego and the Id*.

10. Erikson, *Childhood and Society*.

11. Erik H. Erikson, "The Problem of Ego Identity," *Journal of the American Psychoanalytic Association*, IV (1956), 56–121; I. Hendrick, "Work and Pleasure Principle," *Psychoanalytic Quarterly*, XII (1943), 311–29; Sol W. Ginsburg, "The Role of Work," *Samiksa*, VIII (1954), No. 1.

12. R. Dubin, "Industrial Workers' Worlds: A Study in

'Central Life Interests' of Industrial Workers," *Social Problems*, III (1956), 131–41.
    13. B. Bettelheim, "Individual Autonomy and Mass Controls," *Frankfurter Beiträge zur Soziologie*, I (1955), 245–62.
    14. C. B. Chisholm, "Panel Discussion: Psychiatry of Enduring Peace and Social Progress," *Psychiatry*, IX (1946), 31.
    15. H. Marcuse, *Eros and Civilization* (Boston, Beacon Press, 1956).
    16. Erikson, *Childhood and Society*.

12. TROUBLED PEOPLE

    1. This exchange of letters following Miss Haworth's original reply to W. H. is not without interest:
    "Dear Miss Haworth: I am particularly interested in and sympathetic to the plight of your correspondent 'W. H.,' who has suffered two nervous breakdowns within the past year, which doctors have failed to relieve. Having 'walked through hell' since last October, he is finally convinced his trouble is mental and, although jobless and penniless at present, he is urgently in the mood for psychiatric help, if you can put him in line for it.
    "You cited the National Committee for Mental Hygiene as a clearing house of information on social services in that field, and advised him to write to the director, Dr. George Stevenson. In the circumstances, you did your best, but I'd like to add my comments for what they may be worth.
    "For 12 years I suffered almost continually from a severe case of neurasthenia or anxiety neurosis. However, during the past year the acute symptoms have been fading away until now I am almost entirely at ease. During the illness I tried almost everything imaginable in the way of remedy, including about nine months of psychoanalysis, six or seven years ago. I seemed to make no progress whatever in that endeavor; hence decided to terminate the analysis.
    "As for you, Miss Haworth, I believe you are a good diagnostician, but I sometimes think you put too much faith in

psychoanalysis as a healing agent. To find flaws in personality and the reasons for them is not too difficult; but to change personality traits is a mammoth undertaking. For my part, I believe time is the great healer. I've learned to accept my limitations, get lots of rest, and avoid situations which might make me unnecessarily self-conscious. I believe good old-fashioned understanding and encouragement from one's fellows is marvelous."

S. N.

"Dear S. N.: Let's not quarrel about analysis, but rather look with open mind at what it is—namely, something mankind has undertaken to develop for mankind's good. It propounds no panacea; rather, it cautiously addresses itself to cleansing festering areas of sickness hitherto ignored or supposed incurable. Also, let's agree, as you say, that changing personality traits is a mammoth task. But let's not expect the doctor to do the patient's work on that score. At best, the doctor can only guide and abet his efforts. It's the patient's prerogative to change or not, just as he chooses. He's a law unto himself in that. And by his performance he mends—or fails—himself."

M. H.

2. I am indebted to Dr. Sidney Axelrad for his assistance in the analysis of these letters.

3. Sol W. Ginsburg, "Some Notes on the Private Practice of Psychiatry," *Bulletin of the Menninger Clinic*, X (Nov., 1946), 188–95.

13. THE PRIVATE PRACTICE OF PSYCHIATRY

1. Sol W. Ginsburg, "Some Notes on the Private Practice of Psychiatry," *Bulletin of the Menninger Clinic*, X (Nov., 1946), 188–95.

2. Doctor Oberndorf died at the age of 72 on May 30, 1954.

3. Most analysts make exceptions for an occasional patient who pays "token" fees. One of the social consequences of the costs of our services is the considerable number of gifted

and highly endowed but impoverished young people whose ultimate contribution to society promises much but the fulfillment of which may really depend on our willingness to adjust our fees so that they can get the necessary help.

4. Space prevents discussion of other important changes, such as the use of psychological testing and the development of group therapy.

14. PSYCHIATRIC CLINIC PRACTICE

1. Sol W. Ginsburg, *The Need and Demand for Psychiatric Care among Neuropsychiatric Rejectees and Dischargees* (1944). A preliminary report for the Committee on Psychiatric Needs in Rehabilitation. Subcommittee of New York City Committee on Mental Hygiene of the State Charities Aid Association.

2. Lawrence S. Kubie, M.D. Testimony before the Subcommittee of the Committee on Military Affairs, U.S. Senate, 79th Congress, pursuant to S.R. 107 of the 78th Congress and S.R. 146 of the 79th Congress, pp. 606–7.

3. "We" in this communication refers to the entire staff of the project. The members of the staff were, in addition to the authors, Vivian Barritt, Miriam Pomeroy, Louisa Blaine, and Dr. Raymond Franzen. The last two, as statistical consultants, were largely responsible for the selection of the statistical criteria, the validation of the sample, and all other statistical aspects of the study.

4. New York City Committee on Mental Hygiene of the State Charities Aid Association, *Needs in Rehabilitation of Men Rejected or Discharged from the Armed Services for Neuropsychiatric Disabilities.*

5. Porter and Davidson, "Alumni Appraisal of Psychiatric Education," *American Journal of Psychiatry*, CIII (Jan., 1947), 441.

15. PSYCHIATRIC CONSULTATION IN A GENERAL HOSPITAL

1. I would like this paper to stand as a tribute to Clarence P. Oberndorf, affectionately known to all his friends and colleagues as "Obie," who was in a real sense my first teacher in psychiatry and to whom I owe a great debt, not alone for what he taught me but for what he represented as a man and teacher. I hope the paper itself will illuminate, if only tangentially, the dimensions of the man and his contribution to psychiatry, especially as practiced in a general hospital.

2. Clarence P. Oberndorf, "The Psychiatric Clinic in a General Hospital," *Medical Journal and Record*, CXXI (1925), 426.

3. F. Alexander, "Psychological Aspects of Medicine," *Psychosomatic Medicine*, I (Jan., 1939).

4. *Ibid.*

5. L. Kessel and H. T. Hyman, "Exophthalmic Goiter and the Involuntary Nervous System," *Archives of Internal Medicine*, XL (1927), 314.

6. In 1920, the year I entered the College of Physicians and Surgeons, the entire psychiatric instruction consisted of one hour per week of lectures during the winter session of the fourth year.

7. H. L. Witmer, ed., *Teaching Psychotherapeutic Medicine* (New York, The Commonwealth Fund, 1947), p. 28.

8. M. R. Kaufman, A. Franzblau, and D. Kairys, "The Emotional Impact of Ward Rounds," *Journal of Mount Sinai Hospital*, XXIII (1956), 782.

9. Ethel L. Ginsburg, *Public Health Is People* (New York, The Commonwealth Fund, 1950), p. 41.

BIBLIOGRAPHY OF SOL W. GINSBURG

1932 "The Clinical, Bacteriological and Epidemiological Aspects of Encephalomyelitis," with Drs. Strauss and Rabiner. In Infections of the Central Nervous System, *Proceedings of the Association for Research in Nervous and Mental Disease*, Dec., 1932, p. 262.

1932 "Subarachnoid Hemorrhage," with Drs. Globus and Strauss. *Archives of Neurology and Psychiatry*, XXVII (1932), 1080.

1933 "Pericapillary Encephalorrhagia Due to Arsphenamine," with Dr. Globus. *Archives of Neurology and Psychiatry*, XXX (1933), 1226.

1935 "Acute Aseptic Meningitis." *Journal of The Mount Sinai Hospital*, II (Nov.–Dec., 1935), 165–68.

1942 "What Unemployment Does to People: A Study in Adjustment to Crisis." *American Journal of Psychiatry*, XCIX, No. 3 (Nov., 1942), 439.

1943 The Unemployed, with Eli Ginzberg, Ethel L. Ginsburg, Dorothy L. Lynn, L. Mildred Vickers. New York, Harper & Brothers, 1943.

1944 The Need and Demand for Psychiatric Care among Neuropsychiatric Rejectees and Dischargees. New York, 1944. Distributed by the Josiah H. Macy, Jr. Foundation.

1944 Needs of Psychiatric Rehabilitation in New York City. Privately printed, 1944.

1945 "Problems in Psychiatric Rehabilitation." *Better Times,* XXVI, No. 24 (March 2, 1945).

1945 "Rehabilitation and the Returning Veteran." *Mental Hygiene,* XXIX, No. 1 (Jan., 1945).

1946 "Psychological Insight—An Aid to the Problems of Prejudice." In American Council on Race Relations, Summary on Public Relations Workshop. Chicago, Sept., 1946.

1946 "Some Notes on the Private Practice of Psychiatry." *Bulletin of the Menninger Clinic,* X, No. 6 (Nov., 1946).

1948 "Aspects of Psychiatric Clinic Practice," with Winifred Arrington. *American Journal of Orthopsychiatry,* XVIII, No. 2 (April, 1948).

1948 Concerning Religious Values: A Psychiatrist's Viewpoint. Cincinnati, Ohio, Hebrew Union College, Jewish Institute of Religion, 1948.

1948 Man's Place in God's World: A Psychiatrist's Evaluation. Cincinnati, Ohio, Hebrew Union College, Jewish Institute of Religion, 1948. Also in Hans Herma and G. M. Kurth, eds., Elements of Psychoanalysis. Cleveland, Ohio, World Publishing Co., 1950.

1948 Psychiatric Needs in Rehabilitation; a Study by the New York City Committee on Mental Hygiene of the State Charities Aid Association. New York, 1948.

1948 "Psychiatry and the Social Order." *Mental Hygiene,* XXXII, No. 3 (July, 1948).

1948 "Social and Economic Implications of Mental Hygiene." In Proceedings of the National Conference of Social Work, 1948. New York, Columbia University Press, 1949.

1948 "Troubled People." *Mental Hygiene,* XXXII, No. 1 (Jan., 1948), 4–14.

1949 The Functioning of Psychiatric Clinics in New York City; a Study toward the Prevention of Waste. New York City Committee on Mental Hygiene of the State Charities Aid Association. New York, 1949.

1949 "Social Science and Social Action: Implications for Mental Hygiene," *Mental Hygiene*, XXXIII, No. 2 (April, 1949).

1950 "Mental Health and Social Issues of Our Times." *American Journal of Orthopsychiatry*, XX, No. 2 (April, 1950).

1950 "The Problem of Occupational Choice," with Eli Ginzberg, Sidney Axelrad, and John L. Herma. *American Journal of Orthopsychiatry*, XX, No. 1 (Jan., 1950).

1950 "Some Potential Resources for Community Mental Health." Michigan Society for Mental Hygiene, *Mental Hygiene Bulletin*, VIII, No. 4 (1950).

1950 "Values and the Psychiatrist." *American Journal of Orthopsychiatry*, XX, No. 3 (July, 1950).

1950–51 "Adolescence Is Hard on Everyone." *Child Study Magazine*, XXVIII, No. 1 (Winter, 1950–51).

1951 "The Impact of the Social Worker's Cultural Structure on Social Therapy." *Social Casework*, Oct., 1951.

1951 Occupational Choice: An Approach to a General Theory, with Eli Ginzberg, Sidney Axelrad, and John L. Herma. New York, Columbia University Press, 1951.

1952 "The Psychological Aspects of Eating." *Journal of Home Economics*, XLIV, No. 5 (May, 1952).

1953 "Concerning Religion and Psychiatry." *Child Study*, Fall, 1953.

1953 "The Neuroses." *The Annals of the American Academy of Political and Social Science*, March, 1953.

1953 "On Growing Up as a Jew." *Jewish Center Program Aids*, March, 1953.

1953 Psychiatry and Military Manpower Policy, with Eli Ginzberg and John L. Herma. New York, Columbia University Press, 1953.

1953 "Values and Their Relationship to Psychiatric Principles and Practice," with John L. Herma. *American Journal of Psychotherapy*, VII, No. 3 (July, 1953).

1954 "Atomism of Behavior." In Donald Porter Geddes, ed.,

An Analysis of the Kinsey Reports on Sexual Behavior in the Human Male and Female. New York, E. P. Dutton & Co., 1954.

1954   On Cultural Factors in Casework. New York, National Travelers Aid Association, 1954.

1954   "The Role of Work: A Contribution to Ego Psychology." *Samiksa*, VIII, No. 1 (1954).

1955   "Adjustment: Its Uses and Dangers." *Child Study* (1955).

1955   "The Mental Health Movement: Its Theoretical Assumptions." In Ruth Kotinsky and H. L. Witmer, eds., Community Programs for Mental Health. Cambridge, Harvard University Press, 1955.

1955   "The Private Practice of Psychiatry." *Bulletin of the Menninger Clinic*, XIX, No. 2 (March, 1955).

1955   What Makes an Executive? Participant, report of a Round Table Discussion. New York, Columbia University Press, 1955.

1956   "Work and Its Satisfactions." *Journal of the Hillside Hospital*, V, Nos. 3–4 (Oct., 1956): Israel Strauss Commemorative Volume.

1958   "The Drive for Integrity." *Mental Hospitals*, March, 1958.

1959   The Ineffective Soldier: Lessons for Management and the Nation, with Eli Ginzberg and others. 3 vols. New York, Columbia University Press, 1959.

1960   "Psychiatric Consultation in a General Hospital." *Journal of the Mount Sinai Hospital*, XXVII, No. 4 (July, 1960).